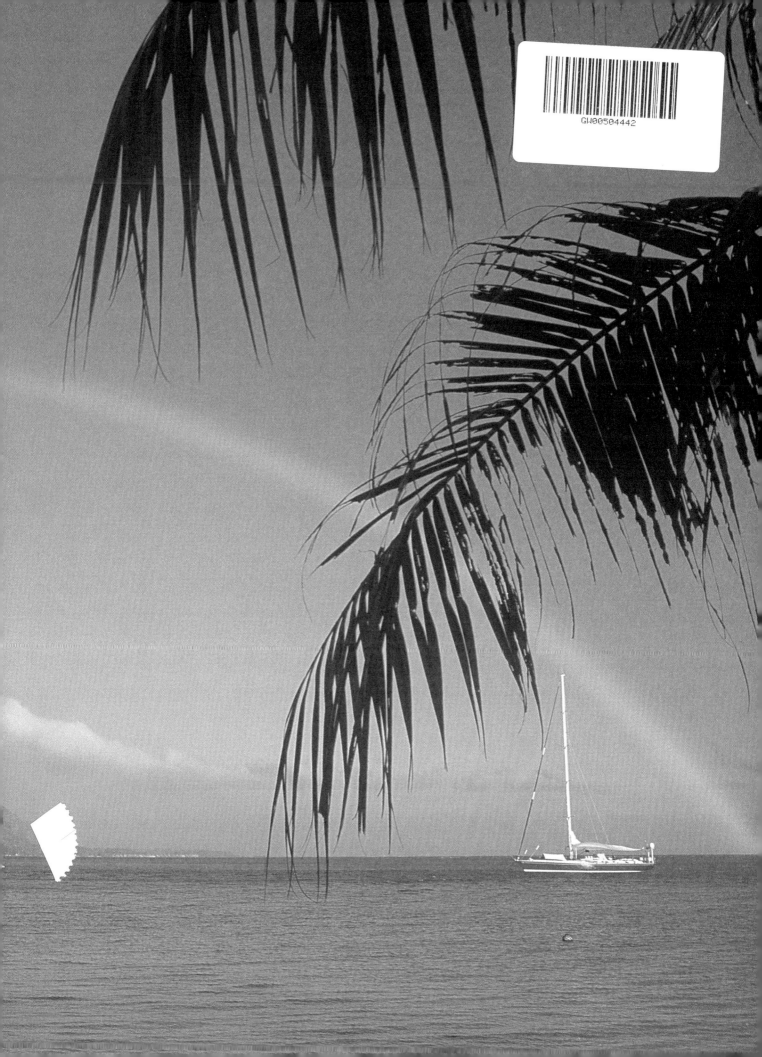

GW00504442

The
YACHTING
HANDBOOK

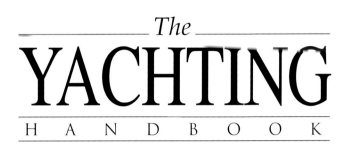

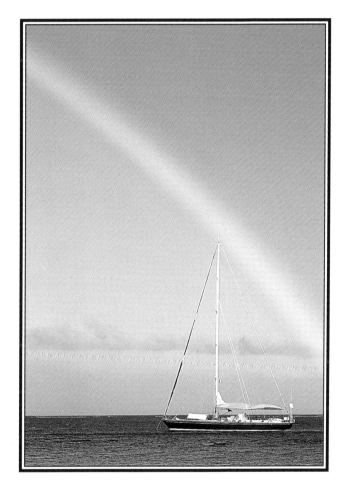

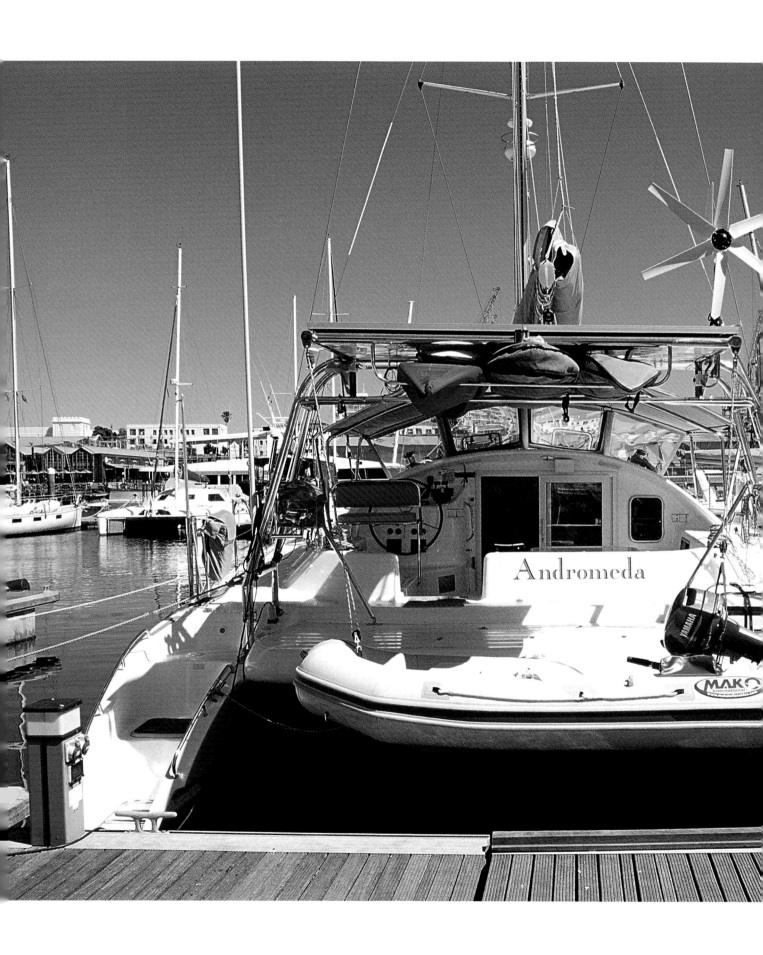

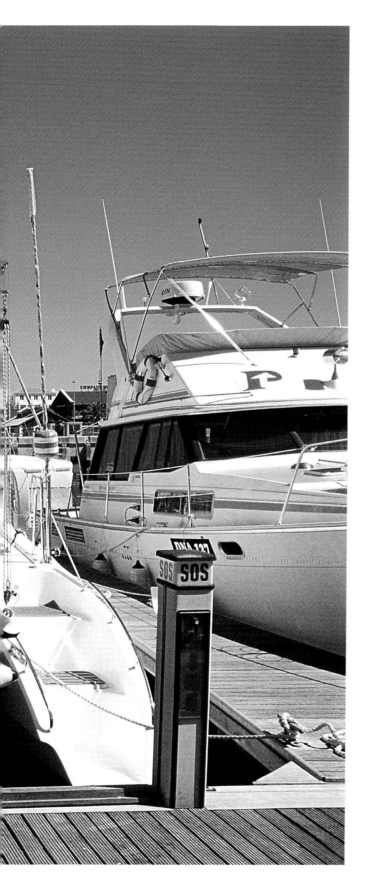

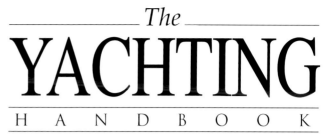

The
YACHTING
HANDBOOK

NEW
HOLLAND

DAVE COX

First published in 2003 by
New Holland Publishers Ltd
London • Cape Town • Sydney • Auckland
www.newhollandpublishers.com

86 Edgware Rd
London W2 2EA
United Kingdom

80 McKenzie Street
Cape Town 8001
South Africa

14 Aquatic Drive
Frenchs Forest, NSW 2086
Australia

218 Lake Road
Northcote, Auckland
New Zealand

ISBN 1 84330 443 0 (hardback)
ISBN 1 84330 444 9 (paperback)

Reproduction by Unifoto (Pty) Ltd
Printed and bound by Tien Wah Press (Pte) Ltd
2 4 6 8 10 9 7 5 3 1

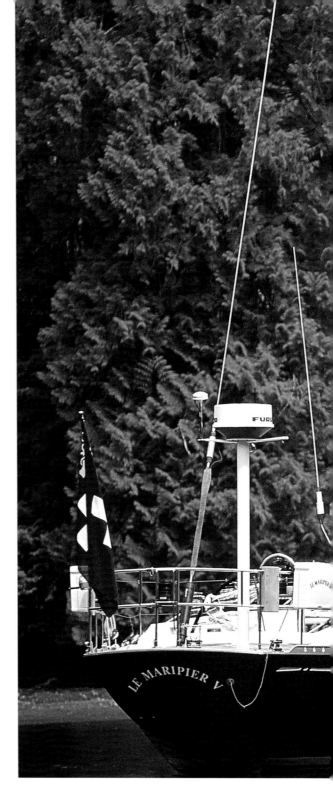

Publisher: Mariëlle Renssen
Publishing managers: Claudia Dos Santos (SA), Simon Pooley (UK)
Designers: Richard MacArthur, Janine Cloete
Editor: Gill Gordon
Illustrators: Dennis Bagnall, Steven Felmore
Picture researchers: Karla Kik, Luke Jansen, Janine Cloete
Photographer: Neil Corder
Production: Myrna Collins
Consultant: Jeff Toghill

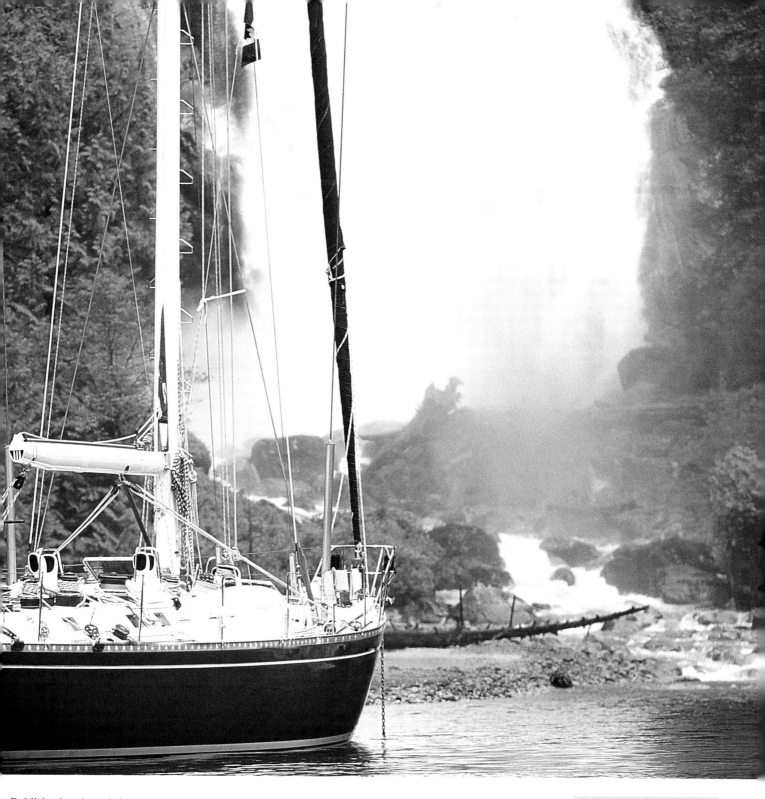

Publisher's acknowledgements

Thanks to Richard Acheson, Acheson Rossa Custom Yachts; the owners of *Andromeda*, Michael Dull and Mary Bradley; the owner, skipper and crew of *African Renaissance*, Gareth Blankenberg, Paul Tomes, Neil McKellar, Marcello Burricks, Neil Hart, James Timewell, Hayley Tomes, Kelly Kieswetter and Robyn Barron; Mountain High Maps/Anton Krugel; the SAN and the UK Hydrographic Office for the use of charts.

Author's dedication

To sailing – for giving me a lifetime of pleasure.

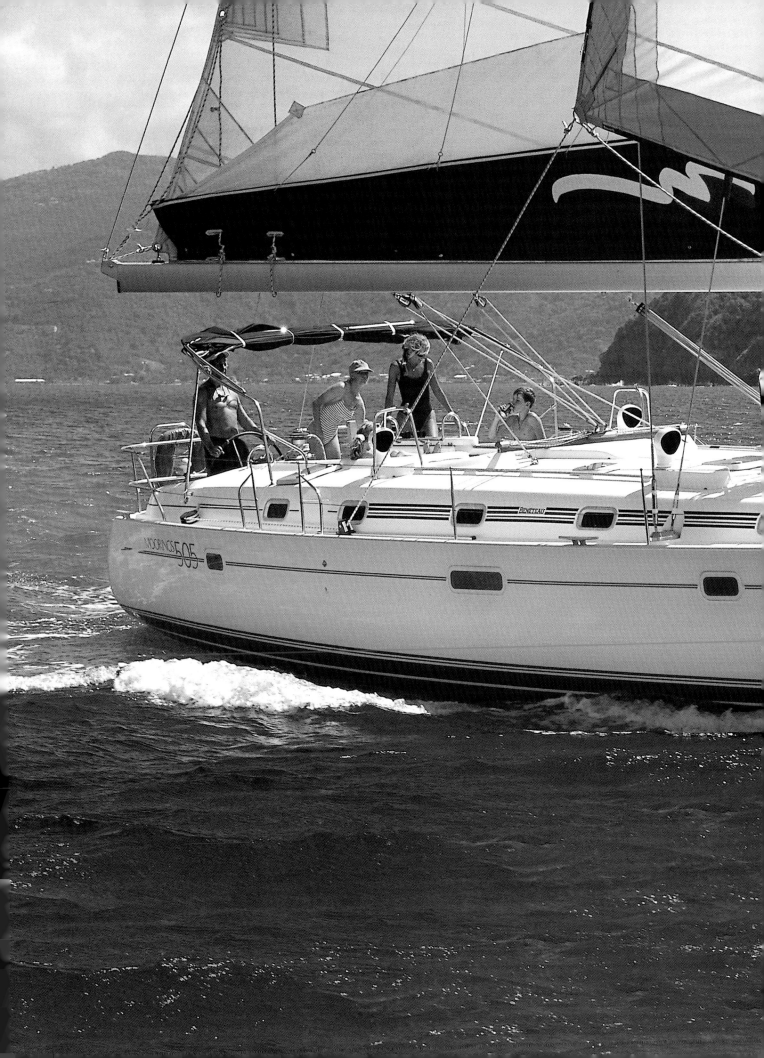

CONTENTS

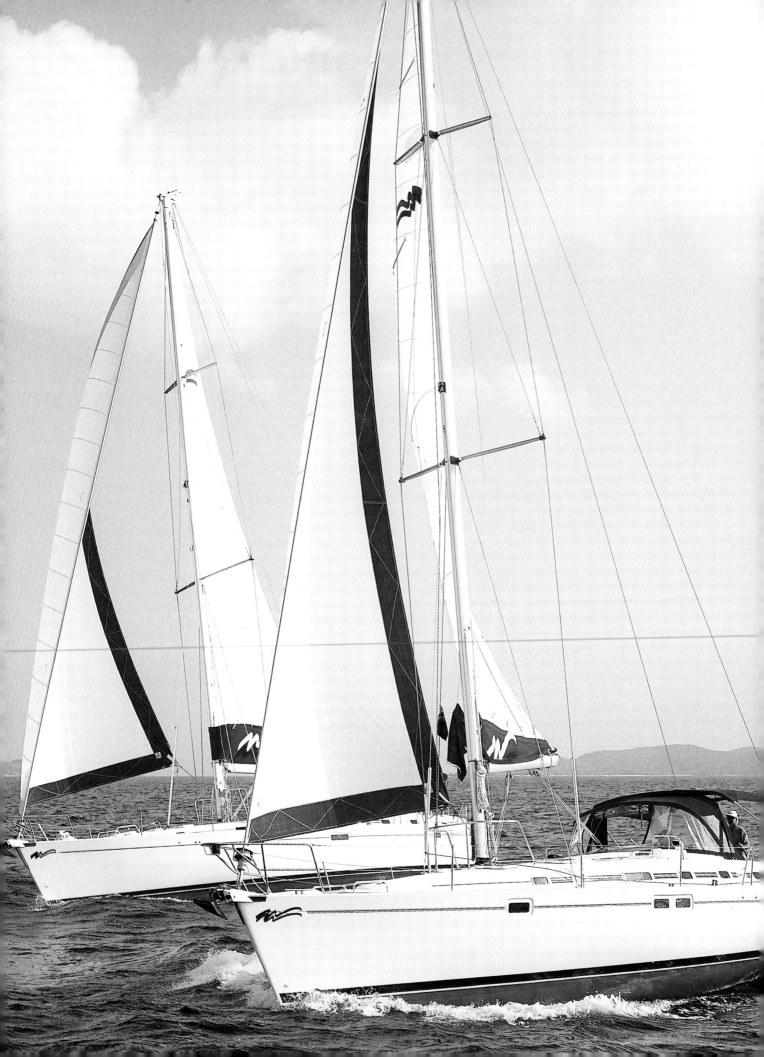

CHOOSING A CRUISING YACHT

This book has been written on the assumption that you have some sailing knowledge and are now ready, or have begun, to test your skills on the open ocean. Owning a cruising boat is a long-term commitment and it is important that you choose a vessel that meets your greatest needs.

Long-distance sailing involves the handling of the boat itself, navigation, seamanship, general maintenance and the skills to cope in any emergency. You can acquire just enough knowledge to sail your boat effectively in the sort of weather conditions you enjoy, or it can become an all-consuming passion, where you continue to hone your sailing skills and learn new things with every voyage you make.

If you intend to do most of your sailing close to home, only occasionally venturing further afield, you might be best off buying a small yacht and opting to charter when it comes to cruising in foreign waters. However, if your aim is to cross oceans in your own boat, your choice will be influenced by your likely destinations. Sailing through the tropics in balmy trade winds isn't as demanding as sailing at higher latitudes (nearer to the poles) in either hemisphere.

If you are going to attempt long passages, you need a boat that is able to carry all your food, water, diesel, spares and gear. Remember, there are no shops at sea where you can buy a box of matches if you suddenly run out!

Opposite Your choice of cruising boat will be influenced by where you intend to sail. Most cruising yachtsmen prefer the trade winds and warm water of the tropics to the howling gales and subzero temperatures of the Roaring Forties.

9

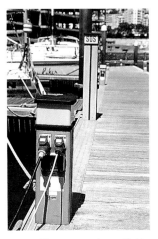

Above *Shore power is available in most marinas.*

Below *A traditional wooden-hulled yawl.*

BUYING A BOAT

Don't underestimate the cost of buying a boat. While a well-built, equipped and maintained vessel holds its value, it doesn't usually make its owner much money. Boat ownership has an ongoing cost, so recognize this and budget for it. Whether you are buying a new or used boat, your choice will depend on many factors, not least of which is the depth of your pocket. When it comes to cruising, size counts, so think carefully about how you intend to use the boat. A small six-berth cruiser-racer is fine if you will make only a few overnight trips a year with a couple of mates, but accommodating a family in comfort for a two-week cruising holiday may require something larger.

Moorings

Once you have made a decision to buy a boat, you need to find somewhere to put it. Start looking at this aspect early on, as some ports won't let you register your craft if you don't have access to a mooring or berth. In crowded areas, like the south coast of England, moorings are scarce and expensive, while in less popular places they are more affordable.

Most sailboats are kept at yacht clubs or private marinas, and the convenience is usually worth the cost. Electricity and water are laid on, slipways and cradles are on hand for taking yachts out of the water for maintenance and there is often a chandlery selling essential repair items. Most also have facilities such as a clubhouse, bar, restaurant and laundromat.

When enquiring about moorings, bear in mind the type and size of your boat. Multihulls (catamarans and trimarans) take up more space and can cost twice as much as a monohull to moor. Draught is a factor in many marinas, although most offer both deep and shallow berths, as well as double berths for catamarans, so ensure you get the right one for your boat. Do your homework before you buy and make sure you have somewhere to put your boat before you sign on the dotted line.

Monohulls

Many monohulls (keelboats) are available in several options, such as a large rig (see p16) and deep keel for racing, or a small rig and shallow keel for cruising. Most production boats, particularly from European builders, are moderate- to light-displacement boats.

There are so many production boat builders around the world that you won't have to look far to find the boat of your dreams. Most production builders work in fibreglass, although some use hi tech resin/glass specifications for strength, or to save weight.

Notable producers include France's Beneteau and Jeaneau, Bavaria of Germany, Finland's Swan and Sweden's Halberg Passey. The USA has many production builders, as well as builders of classic craft made from modern materials, to meet the demand for traditional moderate- to heavy-displacement sailboats styled on older designs.

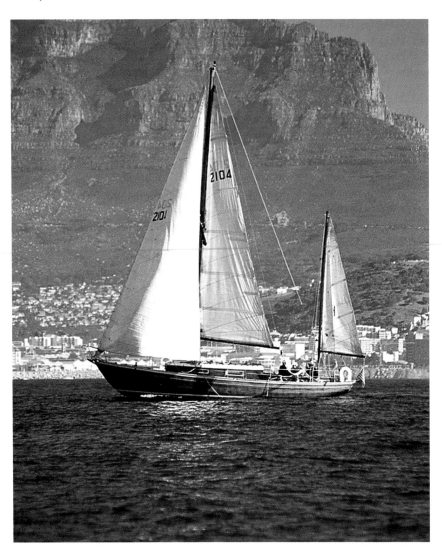

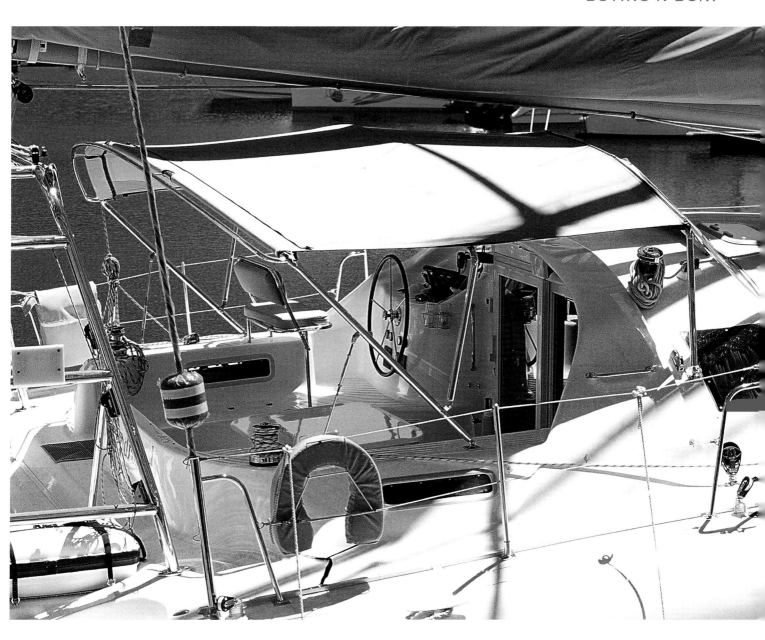

Multihulls

These are particularly popular in the charter cruising market as they are comfortable, stable and don't roll at anchor, a big plus over a monohull. The deck area is usually spacious and the accommodation can easily be divided up for charter groups. In addition, their shallow draught makes them ideal for sailing close inshore, such as in the Caribbean.

International safety rules for multihulls insist that there are hatches on the underside of all the hulls to facilitate getting out in the event of a capsize. If you are buying a catamaran, check this – getting trapped down below is not an experience to be recommended. Despite their tendency to capsize, they are generally seaworthy and, provided they are treated with respect, will look after their crew in bad conditions.

The average cruising multihull does not go well to windward and may need the engine to make progress or manoeuvre on this point of sail. (With a diesel engine in each hull, production catamarans can be considered power-assisted sailboats.) Judicious use of the engines can improve performance substantially.

Above *Big cruising catamarans are spacious and comfortable at sea and at anchor.*

STRUCTURE OF THE BOAT

Hull type and design

Your choice of hull depends on your sailing requirements and your experience. If you enjoy driving a boat to its limits, then performance will be your prime consideration, but you may care more about on-board comfort and easy handling in moderate weather conditions than performance.

For everyday cruising and local offshore racing, moderate-displacement boats offer good performance and reasonable load-carrying capacity. (Displacement is the term for the weight of water a yacht displaces when floating under a normal sailing load – with its standard array of sails, rigging etc.)

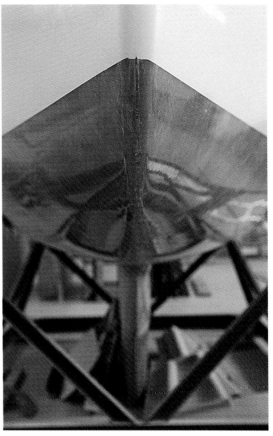

Modern production boats have clean, undistorted hull lines and a good speed to weight ratio. Many older boats are heavy displacement and can pull up a big wake when going fast, but they are capable of making fast passages, with the advantage that they can be heavily loaded without compromising their seaworthiness. Racing yachts are designed to be light in the water to help achieve maximum speed, but this is quickly compromised if they are overloaded.

When considering hull design and displacement, you should take account of ultimate stability – the angle to which a boat can heel (lean over before going upside down) before righting itself. Although a boat should be able to right itself from an angle of 180°, it is generally not possible to achieve this and 125° is considered the minimum safe figure.

Monohulls have better reserve stability than multihulls, meaning they recover better if they are knocked down, whereas multihulls have more initial stability and tend to remain inverted if knocked down.

Opposite *A smooth finish enables a hull to glide through the water with minimum resistance.*

Below *An aluminium-hulled boat is left unpainted so that any corrosion is soon noticed.*

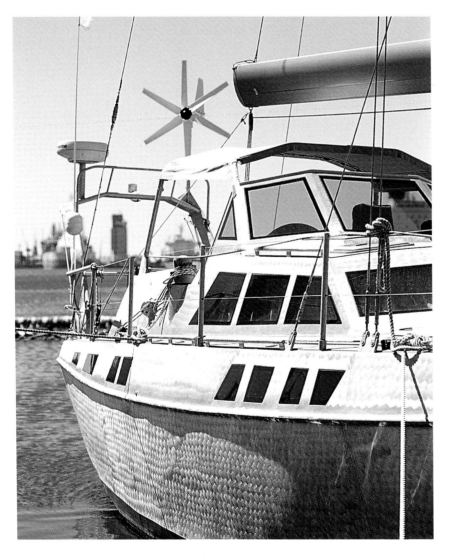

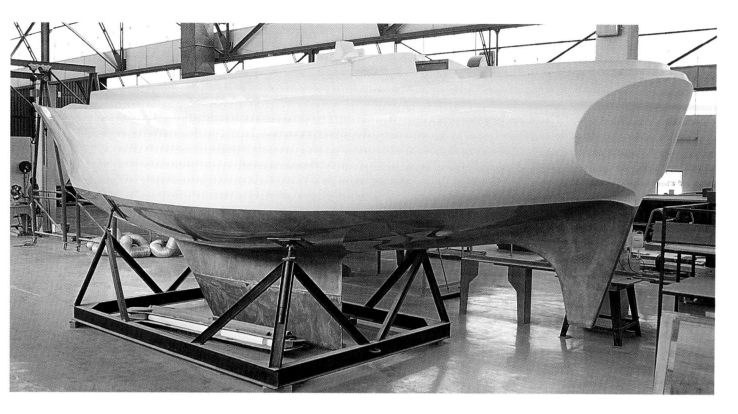

Construction materials

Hulls are built of a number of different materials. Here is an overview of the more common ones.

Fibreglass Also known as glass fibre or GRP (glass reinforced plastic), it is used for the majority of production boats. Comprising mainly polyester resin (some racing boats are built with epoxy resins), with foam or balsa cores. Strategic areas may be reinforced with carbon fibre or a special cloth which absorbs less resin and results in a stronger boat.

With polyester fibreglass boats, you need to watch out for osmosis, which can range from a series of small bubbles in the gel coat to some deep pitting. Osmosis can easily be fixed, but severe cases need drying out before being repaired. A small amount of osmosis would not be a reason for rejecting a boat.

Steel An excellent option for a cruising boat as it is basically collision-proof. The key problem is rust, so upkeep is high. Steel boats built by boat builders are usually one-offs, but it is popular with amateur boat builders. If considering buying from the latter, pay particular attention to the welds.

Aluminium This is a lightweight metal and, like steel, difficult to penetrate. However, the correct alloy must be used to avoid electrolysis, which can be countered by using anodes (see p14). Aluminium is widely used by one-off builders.

Wood Don't buy a traditionally built wooden boat unless you are a dedicated handyman who can cope with the ongoing maintenance! However, if you are serious about owning a wooden boat, inspect it very carefully for rot, particularly in the deck area. If there are any leaks which admit rain water, you will almost certainly find rot.

Wood/epoxy This is a great way of building a one-off boat. A hull is built in wood, often strip-planked in red cedar, and then coated with epoxy and fibreglass. Sometimes the wood is simply used as a core, with a substantial amount of fibreglass inside and out, resulting in a wood-cored fibreglass boat. In other projects the wooden boat itself is structural and epoxy is used to finish or protect the boat. Epoxy adheres to timber better than polyester and some excellent wood/epoxy boats have been built. Maintenance is generally low.

Above *Most modern production boats are made from fibreglass.*

Below *Careful craftsmanship ensures that a wooden ship remains watertight.*

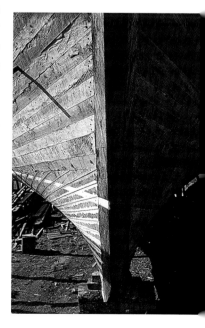

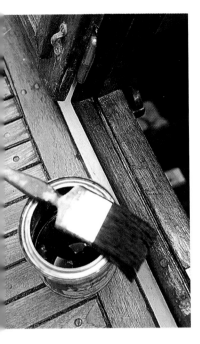

Above *Use marine varnish to seal and protect most wooden surfaces. Teak can be left bare.*

Below *Both the hull and the self-steering rudder should be inspected on your annual haul-out.*

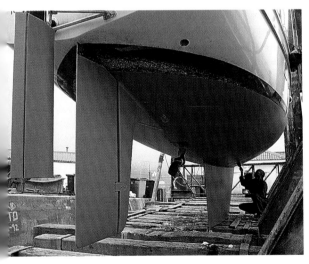

MAINTENANCE

Most production boats don't require much exterior maintenance. Fibreglass hulls have a gel coat which, if cared for, has a long life. Regularly using fresh water to wash off the salt helps to preserve the shine.

Occasionally, the hull topsides (the area between the waterline and deck) needs to be cleaned with a purpose-made rubbing compound, and finished with wax polish – a process not too different from maintaining your motor vehicle. With proper attention a gel coat should last 10–15 years. However, the closer you are to the tropics, the faster the degradation by UV (ultraviolet) light from the sun.

Some production boats have timber on deck. This is usually teak, which needs little or no maintenance. (Bare teak will come to no harm, but it can be oiled or varnished.) Protect all other types of timber with at least five coats of marine varnish.

Construction materials such as wood, steel and aluminium, can be maintained by coating them with a hard-surface finish (such as Awlgrip or International) which responds to the same treatment as gel coat on a fibreglass hull.

Repairing hull damage

Dents in the hull are inevitable and should be repaired immediately. Timber boats are easy to repair if you have woodworking skills. Steel and alloy hulls are rarely penetrated, although they can be dented. Dents can simply be filled, faired up and repainted.

For small dents, the correct fillers and touch-up material can usually be obtained from a DIY store or fibreglass retailer. In the case of major damage however, it is better to claim from insurance and have the hull professionally repaired. Even if the hull has been penetrated (hopefully above the waterline), the experts should be able to repair it.

Electrolysis

Electrolysis occurs wherever different metals occur in close proximity. It is the chemical reaction that takes place between dissimilar metals where an electrical current flows across them as a result of immersion in salt water.

Hulls and skin fittings are particularly affected. Electrolysis can be prevented by using anodes (small plates made from a metal that corrodes easily). When these are attached to the hull, they corrode first, thereby preserving the actual fittings.

There is a scale for determining what anodes to use according to the amount of wear caused by electrolysis. If you are buying a second-hand boat, get a marine surveyor to check for this. It may be necessary to withdraw a keel bolt in order to check properly.

Steering systems

The most simple and reliable steering system a sailboat can have is a tiller, but this is best suited to boats under about 12m (40ft). After that, it gets too cumbersome and the power needed to move it can be fierce.

The tiller is normally attached at the top of a rudder shaft by means of a lifting fitting, which allows the helmsman to stand up and lift the tiller for close quarters manoeuvering.

Most yachts over 12m (40ft) have a wheel that is driven either by a cable connected to a quadrant on the rudder shaft or by a hydraulic system. Wheel systems developed for racing craft can be very sensitive, and a wheel with moderate feel is ideal for the average cruising yacht. (Try to avoid a real 'clunker' of a system with little feel to it.)

Steering systems can and do go wrong, so make sure you know how yours works and that all the components are accessible. This particularly applies to production yachts where there is a tendency to hide everything behind joinery work and panels so as not to spoil the accommodation.

All wheel steering installations should have some form of emergency steering, usually by means of a tiller fitted at the rudder head. Before setting off on a long cruise, ensure yours is in working order and that you know how to operate it.

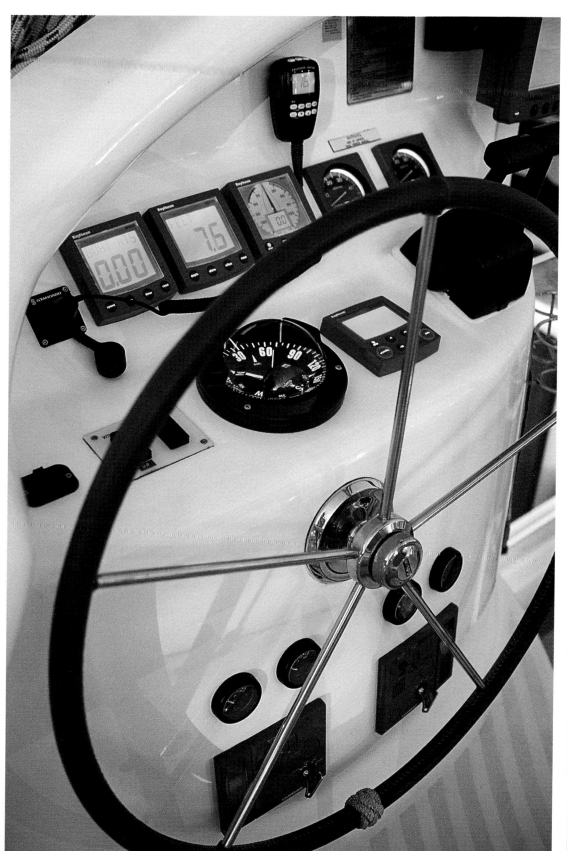

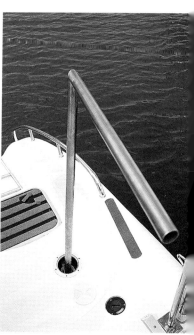

Left *A good wheel and steering system should be responsive and reliable. The instrument console on this catamaran is positioned so that the helmsman can navigate while steering.*

Below *Take time to learn how your emergency steering system works – before you need it!*

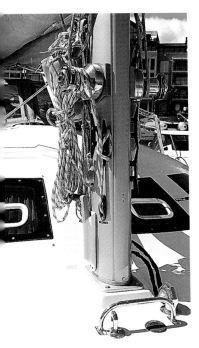

Above *On most production boats, the mast is made from aluminium, which is both light and strong.*

Opposite *Practise hoisting your storm jib in good conditions, so you can sort out any sheeting problems in advance.*

ESSENTIAL EQUIPMENT

The rig

The rig consists of the mast, stays, spreaders and all the paraphernalia required to hoist the sails and hold them in place. Single-masted rigs are the most common, as either a sloop (a yacht with a single headsail) or a cutter (multiple headsails). The mast can have single or multiple spreaders. Running backstays can be a problem to operate when sailing short-handed (with too few crew) and can cause a dismasting, so avoid them if possible. On many cruising boats, the work of the running backstays is done by swept-back spreaders and by leading the shrouds to chainplates set well aft of the mast's deck position.

Modern masts are made of aluminium, although carbon fibre is also popular. Aluminium lasts a long time and doesn't fail very often, but the rigging and fittings attached to it can fail. Stainless steel, which is used for stays and fittings, is subject to metal fatigue which is not easily visible. Standing rigging should be replaced at least every seven years, depending on how often or hard the boat is sailed. Universal couplings (toggles) should be used with rigging screws to minimize metal fatigue. Many dismastings are initiated by the failure of stainless steel wire, terminals, bottle-screws or fittings.

A keel-stepped mast, which goes through the deck to the hull, offers performance advantages. It entails making the aperture watertight and results in the mast intruding into the cabin, but it is able to take greater stresses than a deck-stepped mast, although the latter is more easily lowered for repairs.

Sails

Sails come in many fabrics and types to suit different conditions and situations. Soft cruising sails made of Dacron (Terylene) have a long life and can take a lot of abuse, while Mylar, Kevlar and other hi tech fabrics are mainly used for racing.

Make sure you have a storm jib and check on your ability to hoist it when the usual headsail is on a roller furler. The storm jib should have hanks (rings or hooks by which to attach it) and probably should have

a stay as well, which may be detachable at deck level. A useful addition to the sail wardrobe is a trisail, a small strongly constructed storm mainsail that is used in conjunction with a storm jib.

If you intend sailing in higher latitudes, where storms are prevalent, you will almost certainly sail under fore and aft rig. If you have a roller-furler jib, ensure you have an alternative smaller jib, preferably set on a separate forestay. Your boat should be well laid out and it should be easy to reef the mainsail. You will not be treated as gently in higher latitudes as in the trade wind areas.

Wherever sails or ropes touch something, they will chafe. Change the leads regularly to prevent chafe but if you can't eliminate the cause, move the rope slightly every few days. Keep spare sailcloth on board to reinforce areas of the sail which chafe.

Sails are often stowed in the forepeak, but these berths may be required when you are cruising. Bear this in mind when planning your sail inventory, as your stowage space may be limited.

If you are buying a second-hand boat, get a sail maker to examine the sails and give you an opinion.

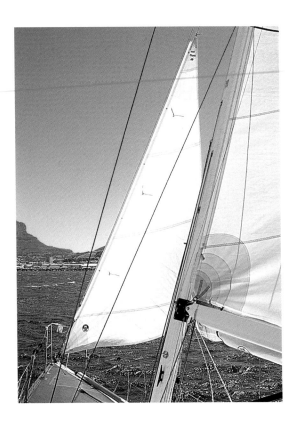

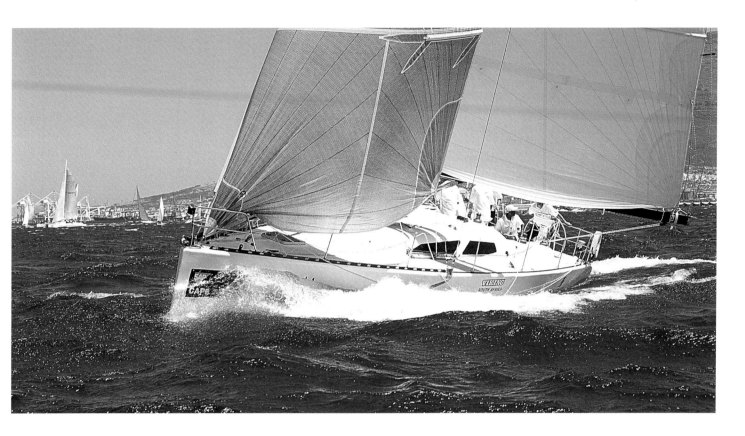

Superstructure

The superstructure comprises everything above deck, including the mast, hatches and coach roof. It takes a tremendous pounding in bad weather and a bulky, badly designed superstructure could give trouble. A low profile is best and cabin tops should be strongly built. Pilot houses have a lot to recommend them, but must be substantially built.

Windows should be small and strong. Picture windows look good, but unless they are made of really thick material they are a weak spot. Consider carrying pre-cut, ready-drilled plywood to cover windows in case they are are blown out.

Deck layout

As the efficiency of jammers has increased, deck layouts have become more simple. Where many winches were once needed, modern boats often have only four winches, assisted by jammers, to handle sheeting the headsails and hoisting the sails, as well as controlling three reefing lines. A well-designed deck layout is easy to operate with a minimum of crew.

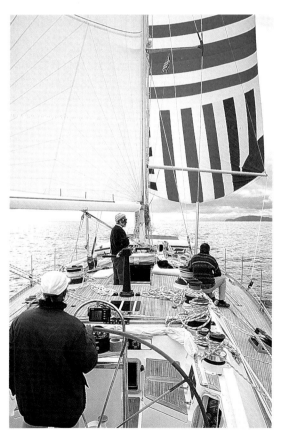

Above *A low-profile super-structure offers minimum resistance and good visibility from the helm.*

Opposite *With a good deck layout, a boat can be sailed from the cockpit, with no need to go onto the foredeck in bad weather.*

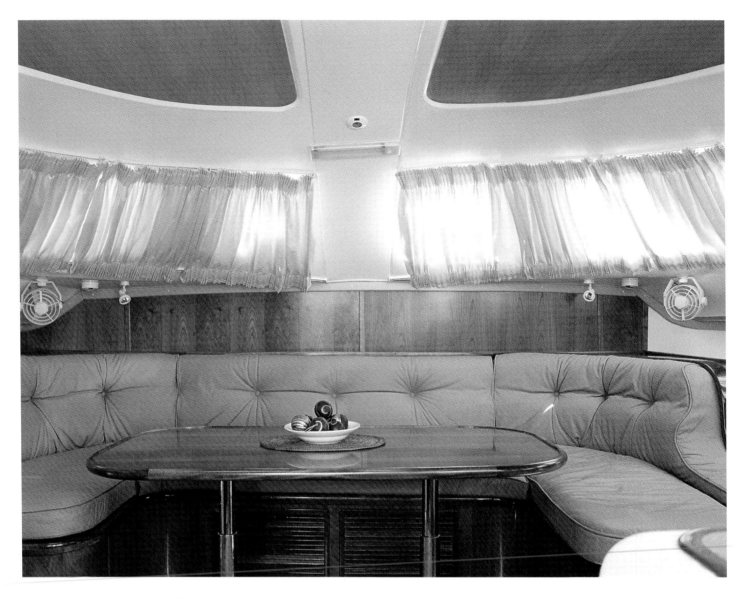

Above *The spacious and comfortable saloon area of a custom-built catamaran.*

BELOW DECK

This term covers your living and sleeping quarters, as well as the galley, heads and general storage. When it comes to accommodation below deck, the degree of comfort depends largely on the type of boat. Small cruiser-racers tend to be functional rather than comfortable, while multihulls that are purpose-built for the cruising industry are designed to be spacious.

If you race, or intend crossing oceans, secure fittings and equipment are a must, but charter boats that rarely make open-ocean passages often have free-standing chairs and tables.

The 'feel' of a sailboat's interior is important. All wood finishes can appear too dark, while only light materials might be too stark. A good compromise is a combination of white or off-white trimmed with wood, which gives a bright, airy feel.

You will probably spend a lot of time down below if you live aboard for long periods, so pay attention to the lighting. There should be enough windows and transparent hatches to allow natural light in during the day, while at night, the lighting in the saloon needs to cater for both recreation and relaxation. The galley area must be well-lit, and each bunk should have its own reading light.

Main cabin

The main cabin, or saloon, should have comfortable seating in a configuration that makes it possible to relax and unwind while at anchor. If you plan on eating meals on board, there should be a collapsible table large enough for everyone to sit around.

As the popularity of bareboat chartering has grown, cabin layouts and equipment have improved considerably. ('Bareboat' refers to a charter boat provided with all food and equipment – basically everything except the crew.) Charter catamarans, in particular, are very well set up. The galley often forms part of an open-plan living and dining area, so the person cooking is not isolated from everyone else.

Many bigger charter yachts, particularly those fitted with inverters, have CD players, TV and DVD or videos for on board entertainment.

Sleeping quarters

On an average-sized cruiser, accommodation is always a compromise. Bunks that are comfortable at sea are often shunned when at anchor or in a marina. When it comes to monohulls, which tend to roll on a long, downwind passage, a narrow bunk with lee cloths is the most comfortable, as there is nothing worse than rolling around in a wide bunk when you are trying to sleep. However, once you are in your cruising ground, spacious sleeping space is often preferable, particularly in the tropics.

Average-size monohull cruisers usually sleep six to eight people (in double bunks forward and aft, plus two in the main saloon in single berths or a double bunk). Boats making long voyages must have good sea berths, to enable the crew to get adequate rest while on a passage. This is not an issue for charter boats that seldom sail through the night, so they tend to have wide comfortable berths throughout.

Because multihulls are a completely different shape, they are less affected by rolling wave movement. They usually have cabins with wide double berths both fore and aft and are generally very comfortable either at sea or at anchor.

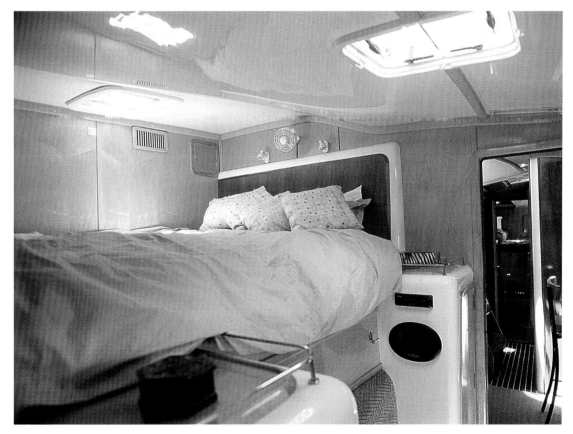

Left *Sleeping quarters can vary from luxurious to fairly spartan. The most important thing is that you are secure in your bunk and will not fall out if the boat heels unexpectedly.*

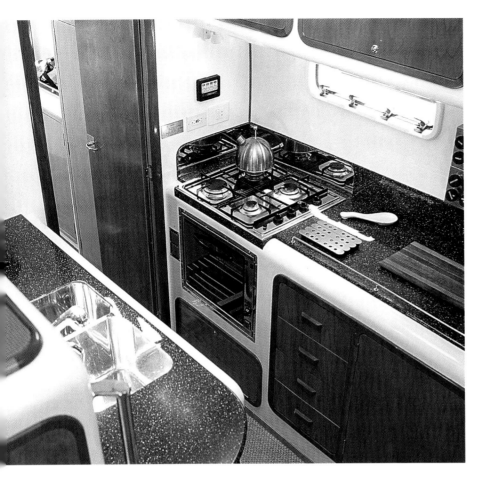

Gas Liquid petroleum gas (LPG) is popular and convenient, but it can be dangerous. Gas is heavier than air, so leaked gas will accumulate in the bilges and can explode when exposed to a naked flame. LPG stoves should be installed to marine specifications, and the gas bottles kept in a separate locker with vent holes draining outboard. The stove should shut off automatically if the flame goes out. A gas sniffer will sound an alarm if there is gas in the bilge.

Paraffin An economical alternative to LPG, and generally easy to obtain. The disadvantage is that the burners have to be preheated with methylated spirits before the paraffin will vaporize to burn.

Diesel Diesel cookers are lit electronically and take a few minutes to get going. The failure rate of the igniting electronics is very low, making them a viable alternative to gas, although they are expensive.

Methylated spirits These look like gas cookers but are completely self-contained. Methylated spirits (denatured alcohol) lights easily and is ready for use immediately. Meths stoves are heavy on fuel, so large amounts are needed for cruising long distances. As meths is relatively expensive, it is more suitable for smaller boats making short passages.

Above *This galley, on a luxury charter catamaran, has all the comforts of a home kitchen.*

Galley

All galleys should have a stove, fridge or cold box and a sink, ideally with fresh- and salt-water pumps. On coastal trips, fresh water can be topped up every few days at a marina, but on long passages, consider using sea water for washing dishes.

The amount of equipment installed will depend on the size and sophistication of the boat. A large bank of batteries, with lots of amp hours, may enable you to operate a fridge and freezer. With an inverter, you can use a microwave oven and an electric kettle.

STOVES

Cooking aboard a moving boat takes some getting used to. In monohulls, the stove should be gimballed (able to remain level when the boat heels) and have movable clips to hold pots in place. A crash-bar in front of the stove helps to prevent accidents and burns when the boat is rolling in rough seas.

Opposite *With a good gas stove and a willing cook, you can regularly wake up to the smell of freshly baked bread.*

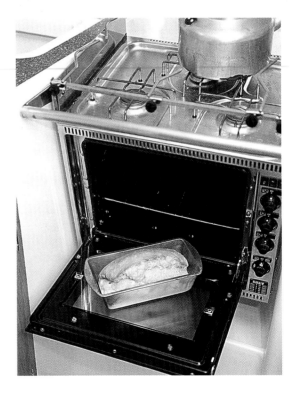

Water systems

On board water systems vary depending on the size of boat and its degree of fitting out. Sea-water and fresh-water taps in the galley and heads are probably the minimum that is required.

Water-makers (which convert salt water to fresh) range from those that produce a few litres per hour to those that produce over 100 litres per hour. Once a water-maker has been fitted, one tends to rely on it, and a mid-ocean failure could cause supply problems. Always have sufficient fresh water in your tanks to get you to your destination, even if it has to be rationed, as it would be a disaster to be without fresh water in mid-ocean.

Bigger or more luxurious boats have showers, with hot and cold pressurized water, which are usually located in the heads (toilet) compartments. An additional fresh-water shower at the stern makes it easy to rinse off after a swim.

If your diesel engine is cooled by fresh water, it is easy to add a carilifier to the system. (A carilifier heats water while the engine is running and continues to provide hot water for hours after the engine is stopped.) Remember that pressurized water is consumed more rapidly than non-pressurized water.

Waste water from the heads, shower, basins and galley sink (known as grey water) may be collected in holding tanks. (Holding tanks are required by law in the USA, where the discharge of sewage, or any other waste water, into the sea is prohibited within a certain distance of the coast.) Many marinas have facilities where, for a charge, you can have the holding tank pumped out.

Preserving the marine environment is important, so find out the regulations for the area in which you intend to sail, and obey them.

For at-sea maintenance, carry spares for all taps and pumps, plus spare hoses, pipes, seals, stainless-steel hose clamps and spares for the water-maker. If you inspect everything regularly, your water systems and heads should not need much maintenance.

MARINE HEADS

Whether your craft is in the luxury category or not, no marine head (toilet) is ever going to be as simple or convenient as the one you have at home. To avoid plumbing problems at sea, all crew members should learn to operate the system properly from the start.

There are two excellent marine heads systems on the market. In one version, which is produced by most manufacturers, a salt-water pump drains the bowl into the holding tank, or overboard, while flushing in clean salt water. The pump operation is controlled by a simple lever. To operate it, push it to the left, and to pump the bowl dry of salt water, push it to the right.

The Lavac, produced by Blakes of England, has a diaphragm pump on the discharge side of the toilet and the toilet seat and lid have an air seal. One simply puts the seat and lid down, pumps the diaphragm pump and a vacuum process sucks everything into the holding tank while drawing clean sea water into the bowl. To empty the bowl, close the water inlet sea-cock and pump it dry.

Both types of toilet can be fitted with electronic pumps which work at the push of a button and both can be installed with holding tanks.

Marine heads have inlet and outlet seacocks and it is important that these are turned off whenever you leave your boat. Many boats have been sunk on their moorings as a result of salt water siphoning in through the toilet. The Lavac has an anti siphon device on the inlet pipe, but play safe and close both valves.

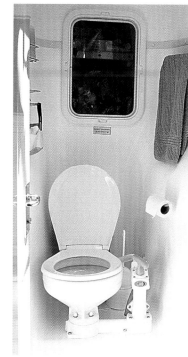

Above *This marine heads compartment in the bow of a catamaran has a shower and storage space.*

Below *Fresh-water-makers, or desalinators, are often found on cruising yachts.*

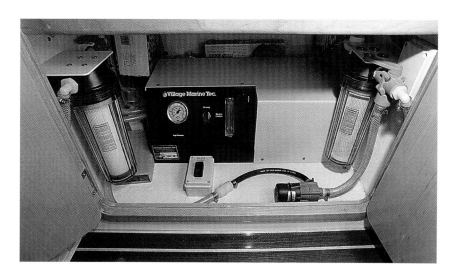

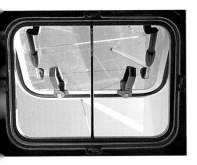

Above *In hot climates, keeping the hatch covers open allows a through-flow of fresh air.*

Opposite top *A heating vent.*

Opposite bottom *An air conditioning/heating control panel.*

Below *Dorade-type vents bring fresh air into the cabin.*

Ventilation

Regardless of the climate, ventilation 'down below' is important, as the functioning of much electronic gear depends on good ventilation. When sailing in the trade winds, you will want everything to be open to catch any breezes. (A chute directing air down a hatchway is a great idea for the tropics.)

Your boat should be equipped with waterproof ventilators. The dorade type, which is universally used, is very good, but make sure you can remove the cowl and replace it with a waterproof cover in bad weather. Many patent aluminium hatches and ports can be left open when in port (provided they are too small for burglars to get through), but they do admit rain water.

When you inspect a boat with a view to buying it, check for musty or damp smells immediately the hatch is opened. There is nothing worse than living in a badly ventilated boat.

Heating

One of the most important requirements for sailing in cold climates is heating for the cabin. Choose from diesel, paraffin or gas heaters and shop around to find the model that suits you best, bearing in mind space constraints, fuel requirements and safety aspects.

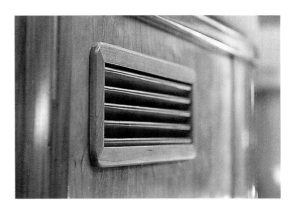

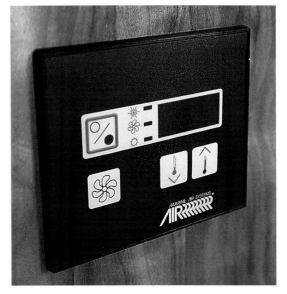

Garbage disposal

Only a few decades ago, most yachtsmen on ocean passages simply threw their garbage overboard, but this is no longer acceptable. Nowadays, all food waste and other garbage must be stored on board and disposed of in the appropriate manner at the next marina or port of call. Plastic and packaging materials must not be thrown overboard under any circumstances, nor must aluminium cans. Recyclable items should be crushed flat to conserve space, if possible, and deposited in recycling bins in port.

Storage

Space is always at a premium on a long voyage and careful planning is often needed to fit everything in. Extra storage is usually provided under bunks and seats, so ensure you know exactly how much space

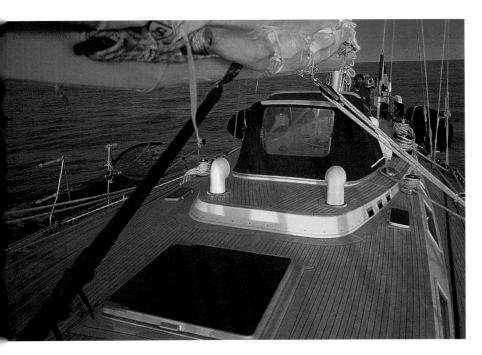

your boat has and where it is located. The galley should have enough storage space for provisions, utensils and cleaning materials. Cabins should have shelves and lockers with some hanging space for clothes and personal items. Set aside one locker for foul weather gear and safety items such as harnesses and life jackets. There must also be accessible storage for sails, sheets, tools and other sailing equipment. All storage should be airy and easy to get at.

Deck lockers, particularly an anchor locker up forward, and watertight cockpit lockers are particularly useful. Cockpit lockers can take the life raft, warps, fenders, buckets and numerous other odds and ends. A lazarette (small locker) aft is also very useful and is essential on some wheel-steered boats to give access to the steering mechanism.

Navigation station

Most cruising boats have a dedicated navigation station, usually situated close to the companionway. The chart table should be large enough to take a full-sized chart folded in half. There should be stowage alongside for navigation instruments, and adequate space for VHF radio, GPS, a sound system and any other electronic equipment you wish to have. It is also a good place to have the yacht's main switchboard.

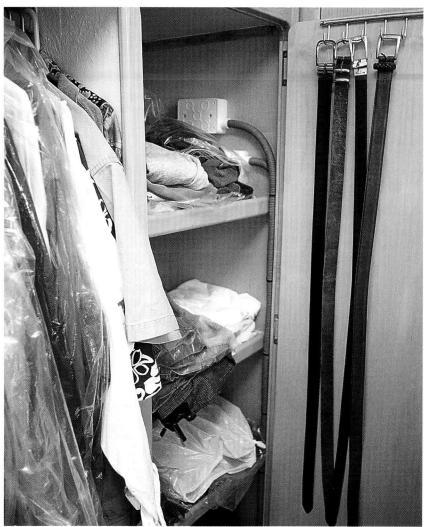

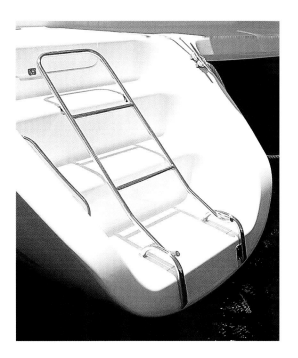

Safety

Sailboats can and do get rolled, so anything heavy down below, such as the stove, should be securely fixed so it does not become detached in a roll-over situation and injure crew members or damage the boat.

Sugar-scoop stern

A sugar-scoop stern or a swim platform is a very useful feature, as modern boats have such a high freeboard (the height of the deck above the water) that they are impossible to board from the water except via a ladder or the sugar-scoop stern. If your boat does not have a sugar-scoop, ensure that there is some means of boarding the boat from a dinghy or for when you have been swimming.

Above *This charter catamaran has a spacious wardrobe, but personal storage space is usually at a premium.*

Opposite *The ladder and steps in this sugar-scoop stern make it easy to board the boat from the water after a swim.*

REGISTRATION AND PAPERWORK

If you decide to buy a new boat from a reputable builder with a good track record, you probably won't go wrong, but get the sales contract checked by your lawyer before signing anything. If you are buying on the second-hand market, it is best to use a recognized broker. Ensure that your offer is 'subject to a marine survey'. Marine surveyors can be found in most ports. They can prevent you from buying a load of trouble, so the cost of a surveyor is worth it.

Registering a sailboat depends on the country, but it is most important to have a document which proves ownership, as you may need it to arrange finance or a mortgage on your boat.

You will almost certainly require the registration certificate if you are going to insure your craft. If you can afford it, comprehensive insurance with third party cover is best. If you can't afford comprehensive cover, get third party cover anyway. A yacht can do a great deal of damage, either to another craft or in the form of injuries to a person or people. Your surveyor's report and your personal sailing qualification will be useful in obtaining insurance cover.

Ship's papers are required for clearing in and out of foreign ports, so keep them safe and ensure you have spare copies made. Buy a file or binder with plastic pockets and put everything pertaining to your boat in it, including:

- Registration certificate.
- Personal radio licence and ship's station licence.
- Personal sailing qualifications.
- Life raft service certificate.
- Customs and Immigration clearance from your last port of call.
- Sale agreement (or your financing agreement).
- Passports of all crew members.
- Crew list, including passport details (have several typed copies of this).

Take this binder with you when you go to clear inwards on your arrival. Ship's papers are hardly ever checked, but you could be in trouble if you don't have them. In addition, should you need the help of your consulate while in a foreign port, you will almost certainly have to prove ownership of your vessel.

SAILING QUALIFICATIONS

Before putting to sea as a skipper, you should obtain an internationally recognized qualification. The Royal Yachting Association of Great Britain (RYA) has a series of qualifications, among them Coastal Skipper, Yacht Master Offshore and Yacht Master Ocean. The American Sailing Association and International Yacht Master Training also offer internationally accepted certificates. Most countries base their qualifications on one of these qualifications.

You should hold at least a Yacht Master Offshore before undertaking any long voyage. The next step is a Yacht Master Ocean, but it involves celestial navigation, which is becoming less necessary now that we have GPS. Many countries will accept an Offshore Certificate provided one has two GPSs on board. In any event, to have achieved an Offshore Certificate you will have had plenty of experience with dead reckoning (DR). If both GPSs go down, DR should get you to your destination.

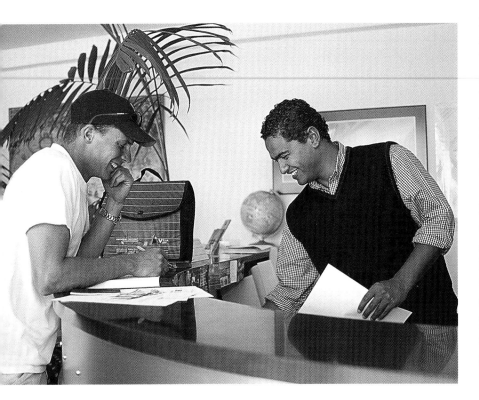

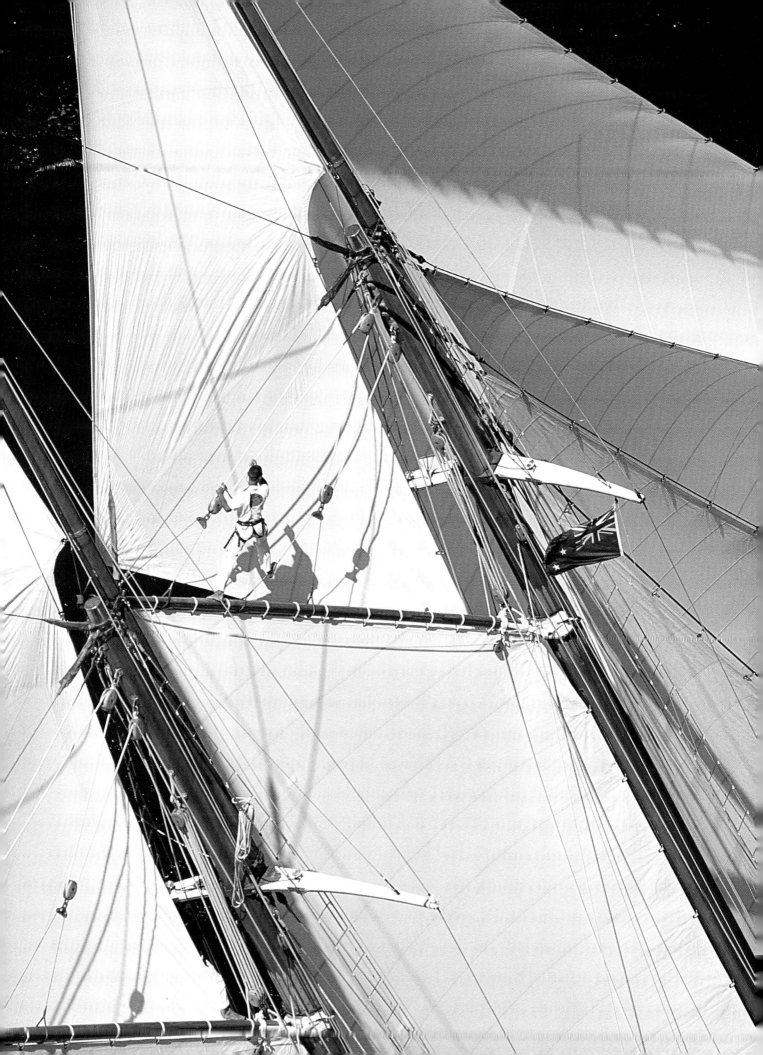

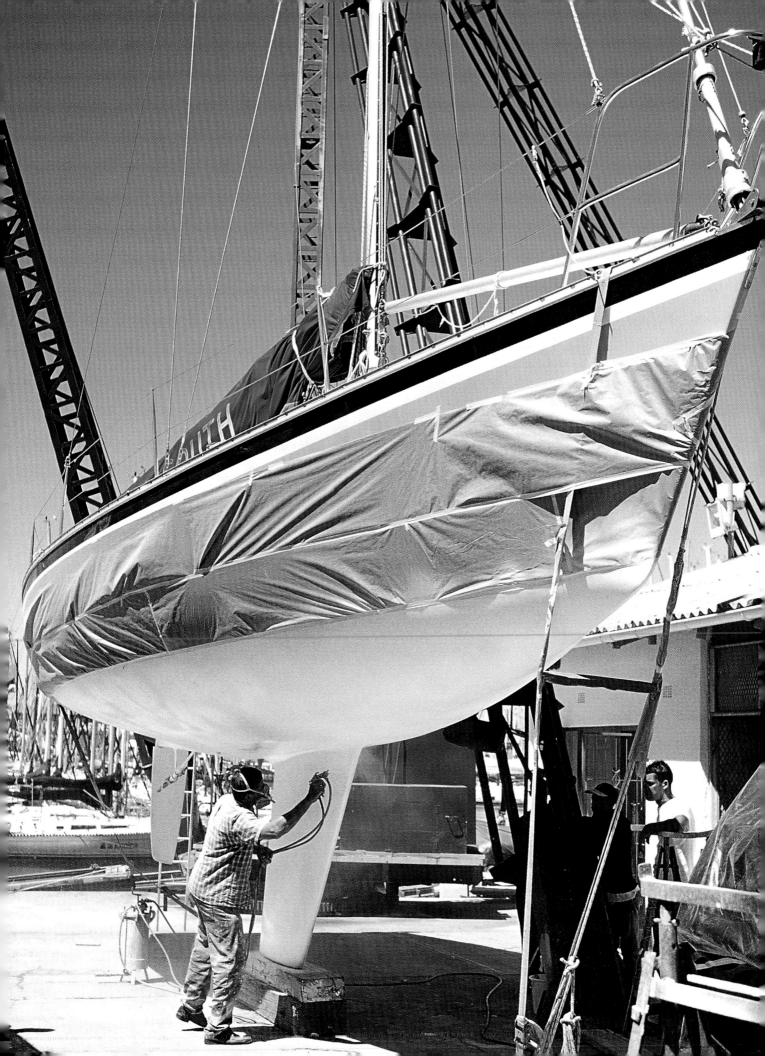

PREPARING
YOUR YACHT

A successful voyage depends on preparation. Perhaps 80 per cent of the effort takes place before the yacht leaves its home port.

There are many questions you should ask and things you need to do before setting out. This is not a definitive list, just an indication what to look out for.

Has the bottom been painted with antifouling paint? Have the water tanks been checked for leaks and are they of sufficient capacity for the needs of the voyage with a reserve in case of emergencies? Has the engine been serviced and do you know how to do simple maintenance, such as bleed it for air bubbles? Are your fuel tanks big enough. If you need to take extra fuel in jerry cans can you transfer it easily at sea? Is your first aid kit up to scratch and can someone on the crew deal with medical emergencies?

Do you have suitable storm sails and have you ever tried using them? Do you have enough chain and rope for serious anchoring? Has your life raft been serviced, and is there a grab bag for it? Is your safety gear up to date and suitable for the voyage you have in mind?

If you continue refining your list and eliminating items then, when you finally depart you will have minimised the risk of anything going wrong as well as put in place the means to deal with any problems. Part of voyaging is the ability to arrive safely without calling for outside assistance.

Opposite *A fresh coat of paint is applied to the newly cleaned keel of a boat that has been hauled out for maintenance and repairs prior to a long voyage.*

Opposite *A crane may be used to lift out the boat for repairs.*

EXTERIOR MAINTENANCE

Hauling a boat out of the water

Before hauling out your boat for the first time, check the equipment that the marina or boat yard will use. Most marinas have a travel-lift or crane that will lift your boat out of the water and place it on a cradle or on the ground where it will need to be chocked up. Find out what lines and fenders you need and whether you need a ladder to get up and down to work on your boat. Thorough preparation will take the anxiety out of hauling.

Most boat yards have a high-pressure water spray that can be used to clean off the bottom immediately your boat is out of the water. If you leave the accumulated marine growth to harden, it will take a lot of effort to remove it, and you may damage the underlying paint layer, which will then require touching up before you can recoat.

Keeping your bottom clean

Every month or so during the year, don a mask and flippers and give your hull a wipe-down underwater (or hire someone to do this for you). This prevents slime from building up, keeps the bottom smooth and will make your yearly maintenance that much easier.

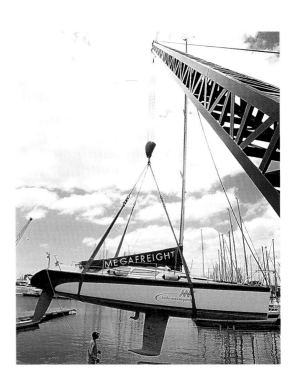

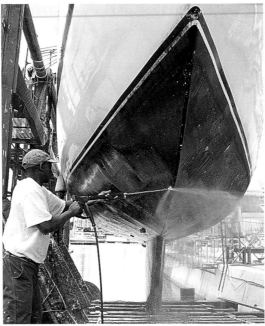

Right *A high-pressure hose makes cleaning the hull easy.*

There is nothing worse than slipping a boat which has never been wiped over and comes out of the water covered in barnacles and weeds. Getting such a boat clean will require a good rub of sandpaper to get it smooth and will probably entail removing paint which will then have to be touched up before any antifouling can be applied.

Antifouling paint keeps marine growth off the bottom of your boat and it needs to be applied wherever you sail. These paints vary from area to area to deal with different fouling characteristics, so choose one that is appropriate for the waters you will sail in. Many antifouling paints are ablative, that is, the surface constantly dissolves or flakes away, leaving fresh paint exposed. Pick the very best antifouling that you can buy for cruising, and avoid a racing antifouling, which is expensive and may have a shorter life.

Antifouling paints used to contain poisons but, with the concentration of small craft in marinas, it was discovered that these substances were adversely affecting the environment and there are now strict controls over the manufacture of these paints.

Antifouling should last for about a year, but if your boat is hauled out of the water for the winter, the paint will only have to last for the summer.

Maintaining the engine

An engine is essential for manoeuvring in and out of berths, making headway in calm seas, generating electricity and, most importantly, to get you out of trouble in an emergency. A marine diesel engine is a reliable piece of equipment and with proper maintenance it should never let you down.

There are two types of engine: a propeller shaft or a sail drive. Most production boat builders use sail drives because there are no lining-up problems and they run smoothly, although they are prone to electrolysis and require regular maintenance.

Diesel engines require electric current to start but, unlike petrol (gasoline) engines, do not depend on electricity to keep them going. There is no ignition system and diesel fuel is fired in the cylinders by compression alone, no spark plug being necessary.

Electric current also generates electricity to recharge the batteries by means of an alternator. Alternator belts are vulnerable to wear, so keep some spares. Unless you carry a spare alternator, there is nothing much you can do if the system fails. The same applies to the starter motor.

Diesel engines are cooled by either salt (sea) or fresh water. In the former, sea water is pumped via an impeller through the engine block to cool the engine. Salt water is corrosive and, over time, can restrict water flow by blocking passages with salt deposits. On rare occasions salt water can eat through the engine block. For this reason, most engines are cooled with fresh water, as in a motorcar.

In a fresh-water system, sea water is pumped into a heat exchanger to cool the fresh water, which is then circulated through the engine. A fresh-water reservoir is marked with high and low levels and must be periodically topped up to the required level. The impellers in the water pumps can wear out or, if the water intake becomes blocked, they can burn out.

A diesel's enemy is air, so make sure you know how to bleed your engine. The operating manual will indicate the bleed points and explain the procedure. In most cases bleeding the engine is an easy task and it could save you coming home at the end of a tow line. Accessibility is important if you have to bleed the fuel

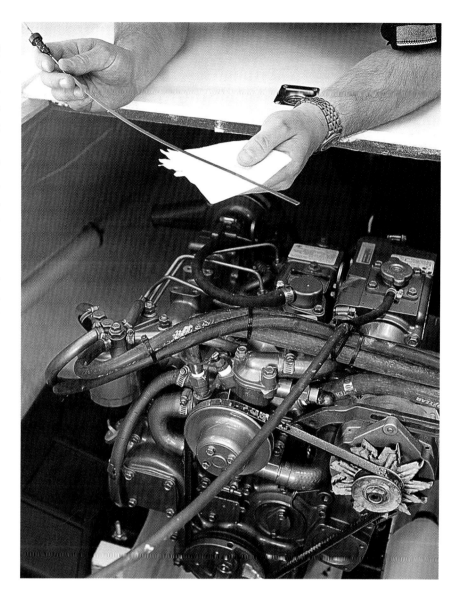

line or do any work on the engine, especially at sea. Engines that are squeezed into tight spaces or behind panels are usually difficult to work on. The engine box should come to pieces easily and rapidly, and the engine compartment should be accessible so that you can get at it to service it.

Keep the engine clean, as it is nicer to work on a clean installation than a dirty one.

Check the availability of spares for your engine. With well-known makes, such as Yanmar, Volvo-Penta, Perkins and Nanni, you shouldn't encounter problems, but always carry extra oil and fuel filters and spares for all belts.

Above *Regular maintenance will ensure that the engine remains trouble free.*

29

Opposite *A fuel filter traps dirt that could contaminate your diesel fuel.*

Keeping your fuel clean

Diesel engines need clean fuel without air bubbles, as an air leak will stop them in no time at all. Maintain your fuel system by making sure that the fuel line is in good condition, all the joints are tight and that the line doesn't snag on any items en route from tank to motor. An additional water-trap filter in the line will remove both dirt and water. Any water present is clearly visible in the bottom of the glass bowl and can be drained off via a small tap, which should be easily accessible. The fuel filter at the engine itself must be kept clean and any air in the fuel line must be bled off at the bleed points.

Change the engine oil and oil filter at the intervals shown in the manual. Most diesel engines are installed close to the bottom of the boat, so there is often no room to drain the oil. A small scavenger pump inserted through the aperture for the dipstick normally does this easy job.

In hot climates, diesel fuel can develop a bacteria known as 'diesel bug' which, if it gets into the fuel system, quickly clogs up the filters and may stop the engine. You can avoid this by buying clean fuel. In addition, using a portable filter at the filler cap will stop any impurities getting through. If you are unfortunate enough to pick up diesel bug, the fuel system must be professionally drained, flushed and cleaned out before you can get going again. There are biocides which can combat diesel bug provided you use them every time you refuel.

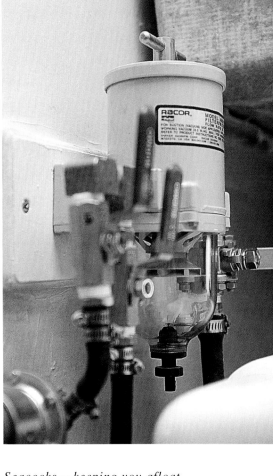

Seacocks – keeping you afloat

On a yacht, every pipe which exits underwater, such as sink outlets, the heads or the salt-water intake, should be fitted with a seacock (a watertight valve below the water line).

The bronze Blake type (shown in the photograph), has the skin fitting and seacock forming an integral part which is almost impossible to break. An alternative is a threaded through-the-hull skin fitting, with a separate seacock screwed onto it. This is acceptable, but it is possible to break the skin fitting between the hull and the seacock, which will cause a leak. `

With all metal components you should beware of electrolysis – the degradation caused to metal fittings by electric current flowing from one item to another (also known as galvanic action). Don't use household plumbing fittings in boats as they will corrode away in a couple of years.

Right *Seacocks allow liquids to drain away. They can be closed tightly by turning the lever through 90°.*

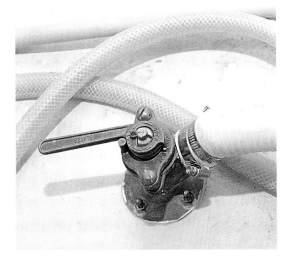

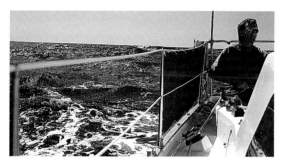

WEATHER PROTECTION

When sailing in very hot, cold or wet conditions, you will quickly appreciate some form of protection in the cockpit area and on deck. Many manufacturers offer various solutions for protection from both sun and wet weather, so choose the best one for your boat and the waters you will be sailing in.

Canopy

A canopy or spray hood over the main hatch or companionway is essential for cruising, particularly in high latitudes. It prevents water from going down the hatch and helps to keep the area down below near the hatchway relatively dry. Going to windward, with spray coming over the boat, it is a godsend. If your boat can't accommodate a full-width canopy, then fit a smaller 'pram hood'. While not as effective as a full-size canopy, it offers significant protection and in bad weather can make the difference between leaving the main hatch open and closing it.

An open hatch contributes greatly to ventilation and wellbeing below decks in heavy weather.

Dodgers

Dodgers, or weather cloths, are lengths of canvas or plastic lashed to the guard rails to protect crew working around the cockpit. If you sail in areas of heavy weather, where there is the risk of losing the dodgers to breaking seas, rather have expendable dodgers than make them so strong that they will uproot stanchions if they are lashed by powerful waves.

Bimini

At sea there is nothing worse than being exposed to a constant burning sun with no place to obtain some shade. A lightly framed bimini, or shade cloth, can be erected over most cockpits without interfering with steering or sail handling.

Opposite *Here, a weather cloth protects the helmsman from breaking seas.*

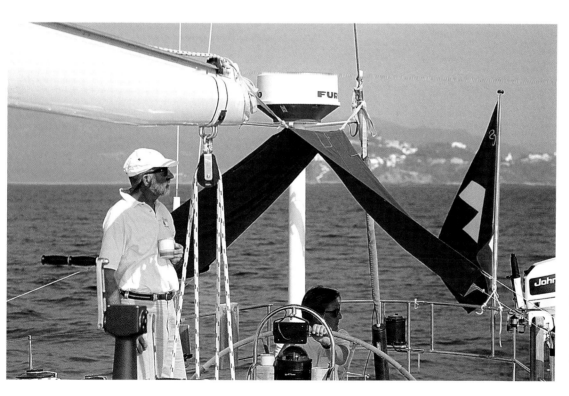

Left *A makeshift shade cloth offers relief from the sun. A bimini is an essential item if you are sailing in the tropics.*

Right *Batteries are often concealed below seats or bunks, but must always be accessible.*

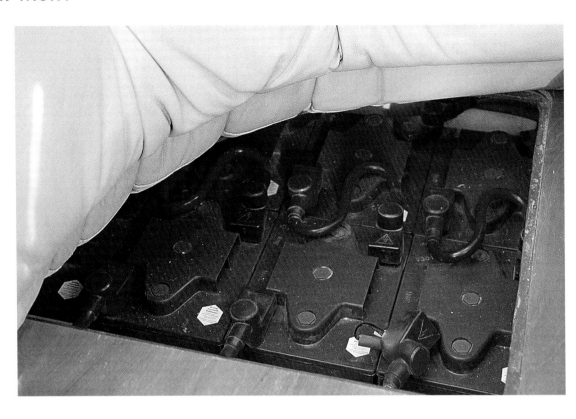

ELECTRICAL SYSTEMS

Batteries

Most sailboats have a 12-volt electrical system (some have 24 volts), usually comprising two or more batteries connected in parallel. Bigger boats require more battery power and an ability to recharge the batteries en route. Separate batteries are used to start the diesel engine and to run various systems on board. They should be switched so they can be used individually, even when the other batteries are disconnected.

The house batteries operate the lights, radios, instruments and so on. They should be high- or deep-cycle batteries, which can withstand many cycles of discharge to nearly empty and recharge. The house batteries operate through a switchboard, consisting of two bus bars (a positive and a negative), from which connections run to a fuse and switch, or a circuit breaker. You need as many switches as are required to service all the craft's electrical gear, plus a few in reserve to cater for gear to be fitted in the future.

Navigation lights should be wired independently, using one switch for port and starboard and one each

Below *An auxiliary engine-driven generator can be used to recharge the batteries in larger boats.*

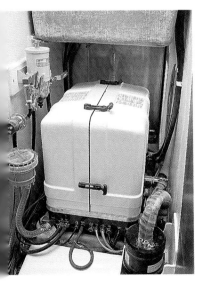

for the stern lights, steaming lights and the tricolour (if you have one). The GPS, compass, VHF radio and instruments should each have their own switches, while the cabin lights could be broken into two groups with a switch for each group.

Each fuse or circuit breaker should be matched to the instrument it is serving. If the navigation light is rated at 3 amps, then the fuse should be in the region of 5 amps. If the current exceeds this, then the fuse will blow, saving the light.

In addition, the switchboard should have a panel for battery management. Most boats have a digital read-out giving battery voltage, amps being used by the ship, etc. If you have a multi-battery setup this information must be available for each of the batteries.

A motorcar or truck battery is no good for marine use except as a dedicated engine-starting battery. These types of batteries are constructed to give a big boost for starting a car engine, but this discharge is rapidly replaced by the engine's alternator, which doesn't happen on a yacht. If nearly fully discharged and then recharged on a regular basis, automotive batteries will fail very quickly.

Charging batteries

The bigger the bank of batteries, the more important it is to keep them charged. One way of recharging batteries is via the alternator of the main engine. Although this will always be wired up for charging purposes, it is not the most efficient way of charging a number of batteries, particularly while in port. Alternators work through a regulator which regulates the current charging the battery. Overcharging or charging at too high a rate doesn't do a battery any good, but devices known as smart chargers allow the alternator to put in a far higher charge, dramatically reducing charging times, as they are programmed to reduce the charge when the battery nears its fully charged condition.

Another option is a charging engine, a small diesel-fuelled unit used especially for recharging batteries, which operates efficiently on very little fuel.

Solar panels and wind or water generators use natural energy to generate small amounts of electricity at low cost. This is normally not sufficient to replenish the batteries of a boat with all mod cons, but is useful for keeping batteries topped up.

Wind generators can be very noisy, although they have the advantage of working anytime there is a breeze blowing. Their noise is not consistent, as it increases in the gusts and drops off rapidly in the lulls. It can keep a light sleeper awake and won't endear you to your neighbours in the marina.

Water generators only work when the boat is moving and are not popular as wind or solar generators.

Shore power and inverters

When you are tied up at a commercial marina you will probably use shore power. Boats can easily be made shore-power-compatible (the voltage will depend on where the craft will be used). You will need a separate switchboard for the AC shore power circuit as opposed to the 12-volt DC ship's circuit.

When you are not on shore power, an inverter will enable you to use a television, microwave oven, some fridges, etc, by converting the 12 volts of your battery system to 240 or 120 volts. An inverter is heavy on batteries, so if you operate one, be prepared to charge your batteries often and for fairly long periods.

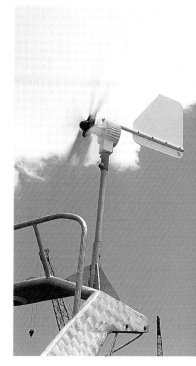

Above *A wind generator is handy for recharging batteries, but can be very noisy.*

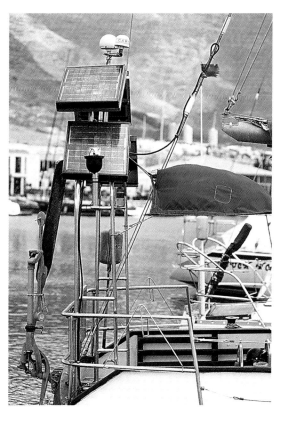

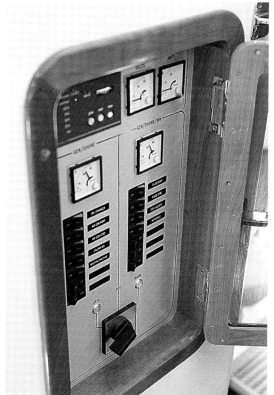

Left *An indicator panel will enable you to monitor the status of your batteries, lights and other electrical items.*

Opposite *Solar panels are a popular and effective means of keeping batteries topped up when at sea.*

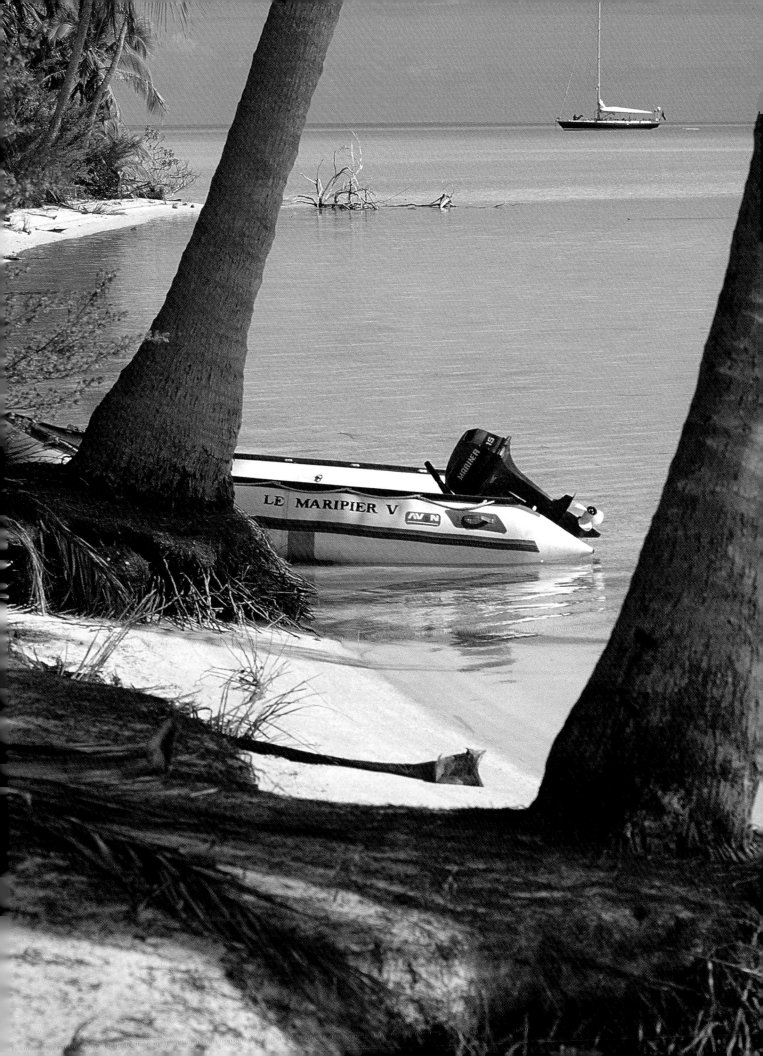

ANCHORING AND GOING ASHORE

When you are cruising, it is essential that dropping and recovering the anchor is easy. You should have two or more anchors that are easy to deploy at a moment's notice, at least one of which should be attached to a rode (the term for an anchor line) consisting entirely of chain.

Anchors should be an adequate size for the boat. One should be permanently mounted at the bow and the other stowed in an anchor locker. A manual or electric windlass and capstan in the forepeak makes it easy to recover the anchor, even if sailing short-handed.

Going ashore

A tender is essential if you will be cruising in parts of the world where mooring is by means of anchors or buoys. Without some means of getting ashore you will not be able to explore, reprovision the boat, or enjoy some time on land.

The most common type of tender, a rigid-bottomed inflatable rubber dinghy, is ideal if you have the space to stow it. Next best is a collapsible soft-bottomed inflatable dinghy which takes up a minimum amount of space. Both types are propelled by a small outboard engine, which requires fuel (normally petrol and oil). Carry this in separate jerry cans, stored in a lazarette or deck locker, separated from the main hull if possible. Stow the outboard engine in an upright position in the same locker.

The tender should have oars and rowlocks (oarlocks) for emergency use, although rubber dinghies are notoriously difficult to row as they bounce about so much and are literally at the whim of the wind and water when you try to row them.

A 'hard' dinghy is very useful if you have a place to stow it. Many convert into sailing dinghies, which can be used to explore shallow waters. Make sure a hard dinghy has evenly distributed built-in buoyancy chambers, so that it floats and will support its crew if flooded. A hard dinghy can be built in two halves for easy stowage. The halves are simply bolted together to give a usable, safe boat.

Selecting a good anchorage

If you are anchoring in uncertain conditions you need to be absolutely sure your gear will hold. Before dropping anchor, check the chart or pilot for the area for any comments on the sea bottom, such as the presence of reefs, wrecks and underwater cables. Ascertain the depth of the water from the chart and turn on your depth sounder while anchoring. Take chart warnings seriously and, if the holding ground appears to be poor, either find another anchorage or be prepared to extend your rode to five times the depth of water.

No matter how tempting the location, never drop anchor over coral reefs, as the damage done to the fragile ecosystem by heavy chains and anchors can take decades, even centuries, to recover. It is better to move on than to damage the environment.

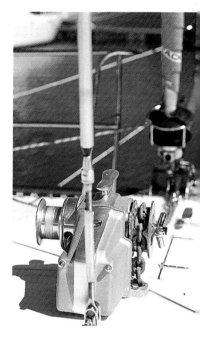

Above *An electric windlass takes the strain out of hauling up the anchor.*

Opposite *Finding a secure mooring means you can go ashore with peace of mind.*

THE CATENARY EFFECT

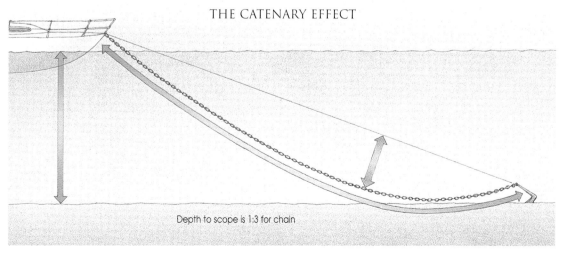

Depth to scope is 1:3 for chain

Left *To be effective, an anchor needs to lie flat on the sea bed. It can only do this if the rode hangs in a curve. This curve, or catenary effect, is caused by the weight of the chain between the boat and anchor, and must be preserved even when the wind and tide are pushing the boat backwards.*

35

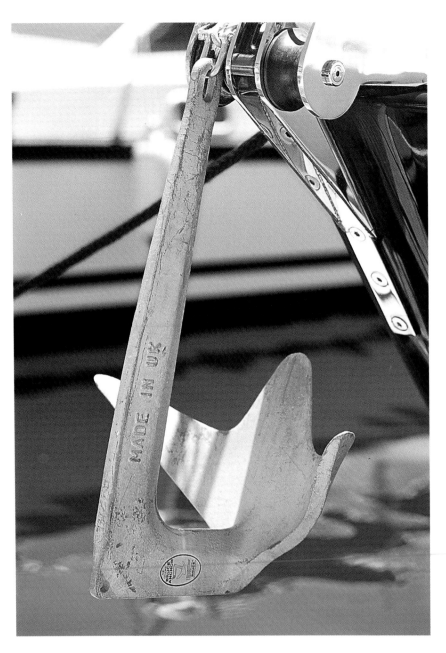

Above *A Bruce anchor holds well in a variety of grounds, making it popular with cruising yachts.*

the desired scope has been paid out, a light kick astern on the engine should be sufficient to bed the anchor. Select two or three prominent landmarks relative to your position and look at them now and again to check whether you are dragging anchor.

Although anchoring under sail is not difficult, it is not recommended in a crowded anchorage. In open waters, you should approach your anchoring position upwind and luff up, stopping as close as possible to your chosen position. Drop the anchor, lower the sails and let the boat drift back.

PAYING OUT THE RODE

The length of rode paid out plays a major role in safe anchoring. An all-chain rode should be at least three times the depth of the water, and a nylon rode should be five times the depth of the water.

An offshore cruiser of about 10m (35ft) or longer should carry two anchors, one with a rode that consists entirely of chain; the second with 20–30m (65–100ft) of chain attached to a nylon rode.

Gravity ensures that the heavy chain hangs down in a curve (see illustration on p35). As tides, high seas or wind buffet the boat it is free to move, taking up (or reducing) the catenary (the curve formed by the chain hanging freely between two points), and minimizing the snubbing effect. Snubbing happens when the boat is brought up with a jerk on its anchor or mooring lines, but stretchy nylon lines or a chain rode help absorb the shock. A nylon anchor rode achieves the same effect by stretching.

Chafing can occur where the lead from a nylon rode passes over the fairlead or bow roller. Use a piece of split plastic hose or a rolled-up cloth to protect the rode from chafing.

The 'bitter end' refers to the very end of the anchor rode. This must be made fast permanently so the end of the rode is not inadvertently paid over the side.

TRIPPING LINE

Anchors can become entangled with something on the sea bottom and have to be abandoned. A tripping line tied to a hole in the bottom of the anchor can help solve this problem. The line can have a buoy on it for

Anchoring procedure

If you are under power, approach your anchoring position upwind. (If the tide is the prominent factor, approach against the tide.) When you reach the desired position, check the depth of the water and drop your anchor, making sure you have enough swinging room for a change in tide or wind direction without getting in the way of your neighbours.

Once the anchor has been dropped, let the boat drift astern while paying out the anchor rode. When

recovery or, if you are worried about the buoy being cut adrift by other traffic in a busy harbour, the tripping line can be taken back to your boat.

If the anchor cannot be dislodged by normal means, motor past it and try to winch it in on the tripping line. Often a pull in a different direction will free the anchor.

Types of anchor

When you select an anchor, choose what will best suit your boat, as well as the type of anchorage you expect to encounter.

Plough (CQR) A good all-rounder that works well in sand, mud and soft-bottom soils. It has a fairly large fluke area, making it cumbersome to stow, but is popular stowed in a purpose-designed bow fitting. It is chosen by many cruisers as their primary anchor.

Danforth Another anchor with big flukes which pivot about the shank. It holds well, particularly in a soft bottom and stows flat, but is not as handy in a bow stowage (where the CQR excels). It is a popular second anchor.

Bruce This one-piece casting is easily recognizable from its two curved horns which help the main fluke bury itself. The Bruce anchor is popular with cruising yachts as it holds well.

Fisherman (Admiralty) This is the familiar, traditionally shaped anchor. It is relatively inexpensive and stores flat, so the stock (cross arm) needs to be unfolded before use. The holding power is not as good as a Bruce, Plough or Danforth anchor, unless anchoring in weed.

Spade An innovative one-piece lead-weighted model that beat all others in tests held in the UK in 2002. Consider it for one of the anchors on your boat.

There are also a number of patent (brand name) anchors, mostly based on the Danforth. Made from aluminium, they are light, non-rusting, easy to stow as they come to pieces, and have parts that can easily be replaced. Although they don't seem heavy enough to hold a sailboat in severe conditions, the manufacturers' tests have frequently achieved better results than traditional anchors. Bulldog (Italy), Fortress (USA) and Vetus (Holland) are three of the brands available.

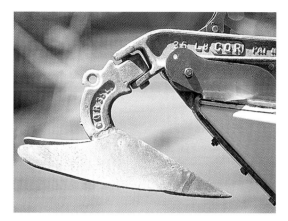

A Plough (CQR) anchor on a bow-fitting.

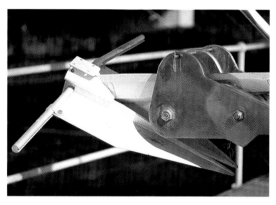

Danforth anchor.

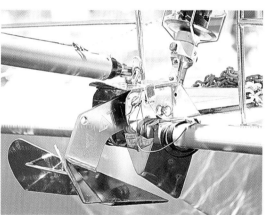

Another type of Plough anchor.

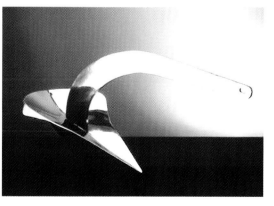

Spade anchor.

COMMUNICATIONS AND NAVIGATION

Most sailors learn navigation in theory before putting it into practice at sea. One of the first things to remember is that what you can do in the comfort of a classroom or at home is very different from what you can achieve at the navigation station on a tossing sailboat.

A cruising yacht needs a workable navigation station with a table that takes a full-size chart folded in half and fiddles high enough to prevent items from sliding off. (Fiddles are strips of wood surrounding a navigation or saloon table. They don't always do the job properly, as most sailors know!)

Be ready to fall back on the basics if your electronics fail and always have on board the simple tools of navigation, such as parallel rules, dividers and a pencil, so you can find your position regardless of battery power or the state of your electronics. Where possible, carry backup electronic equipment, such as a hand-held, waterproof VHF radio and GPS, in addition to the boat's main set.

Always keep a log (a descriptive record of your voyage), no matter how simple it is. Logging barometric pressure, wind strength and direction, boat speed and GPS position every hour is easy to do and, if you don't want to write a more detailed log, you will still have a basic record.

You should carry charts for areas adjacent to your proposed cruising ground so that if your plans change, or you encounter bad weather, you have information on alternative ports and routes. There is nothing worse than trying to enter a port for which you don't have adequate information.

Opposite *The ability to navigate safely is vital in coastal waters, particularly when fog limits visibility to a few metres.*

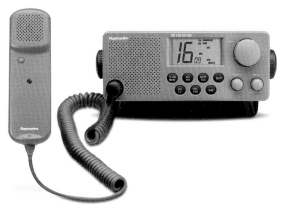

COMMUNICATIONS AT SEA

Regular sailing communications include informing coastal authorities of your movements, obtaining clearance to enter or leave a port and getting details of weather and sea conditions, all of which is usually accomplished via a marine radio.

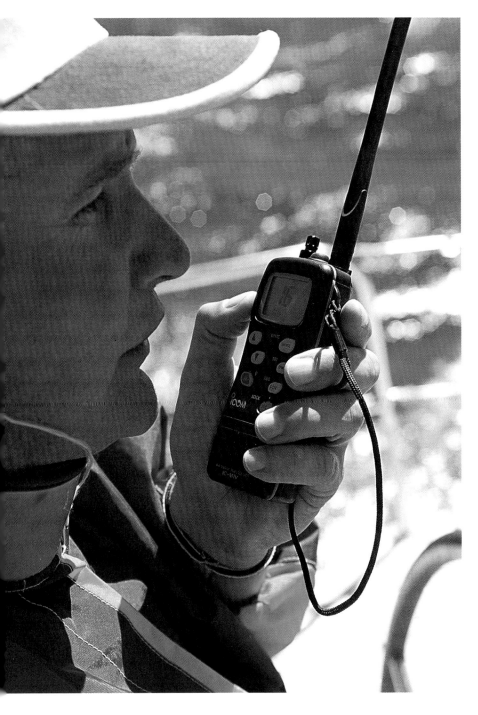

VHF radio

All modern sailboats are fitted with VHF radio. It operates at short range and in line of sight, so it is possible to use the same frequencies without interference in ports as little as 45–65km (30–40 miles) apart. If your aerial is in sight of the station to which you are transmitting, you should get through. There are very few atmospherics with VHF and voice is normally crystal-clear. As one gets out of range the signal starts breaking up, until nothing more can be heard via that transmitting station.

A VHF radio must be fitted before other radio equipment. It can be used to contact port authorities, marinas and coastal radio stations, which will patch phone calls through to you. Depending on the laws of your country of registration, you may require a ship's station radio licence for the set and a VHF operator's licence for yourself, both of which are relatively simple to obtain.

The main calling frequency on VHF is channel 16. After making initial contact, you will move to one of the working frequencies internationally designated for communication by port authorities or for radio-telephone and inter-ship operations.

Installing a VHF is very simple: put it in, connect it to the antenna (aerial), connect it to 12-volt power, switch it on and it should work.

It is a good idea to have a second, waterproof, hand-held VHF on board, to be taken on a life raft in an emergency, or used in the unlikely event of the main set failing.

SSB radio

The number of coastal radio stations able to receive SSB (single sideband transmission) radio-telephone calls is diminishing and SSB is frequently said to be on its way out due to widespread satellite communications. However, throughout the world, radio hams (amateur operators) run a network which gives marine information and weather forecasts. They also talk to sailboats with ham licences. You will barely have left an area covered by one ham network before you enter the next and it is a great way to get weather information and be kept in touch.

SSB operates on both marine and ham frequencies, but to get the benefit of both you will need a marine ship's station licence and a ham licence. If unblocked, most marine sets will operate on ham frequencies and most ham sets will operate on marine frequencies. If you have both an SSB marine operator's licence and a ham licence, then the radio licensing authorities in your country may license your marine or ham set for both purposes.

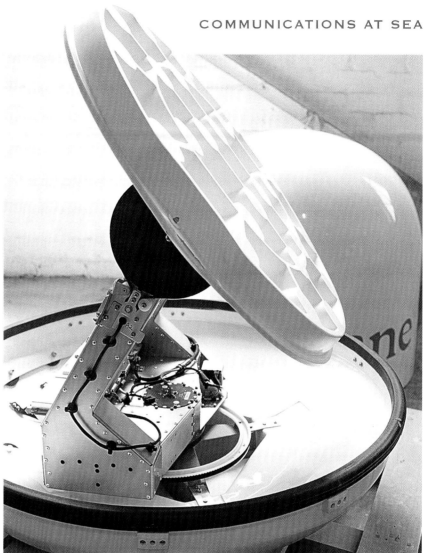

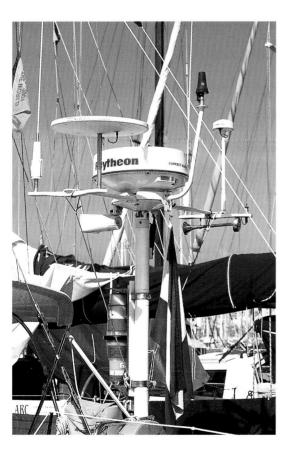

Mobile and satellite phones

As areas of coverage expand, mobile (cell) phones are being used increasingly by sailors cruising in coastal waters. Satellite telephony is extending things even further, so now even open-ocean sailors can communicate with relative ease.

The Iridium system provides a worldwide satellite telephone network that operates in a similar manner to a mobile phone: you buy a handset, sign up with a service provider and away you go. Contact is easy, direct and one usually gets through. The cost of the instrument is not huge as marine communications go, but call charges are fairly high. There are other satellite phones on the market, but most don't have the worldwide coverage of the Iridium network, making it a good choice for ocean crossings.

Above *A satellite dome with the cover removed, showing its internal workings.*

Opposite *Large modern yachts are often bristling with all the antennae required by satnav communications.*

Satellite systems

Satellite communications systems provide a means to send and receive communications, and to notify the appropriate authorities of an emergency situation. The many systems available include the following:

Satcom C/Inmarsat C This relatively compact receiving and transmitting system allows both e-mail and fax messages to be sent and received from anywhere in the world.

International SOLAS (Safety of Life at Sea) regulations require Inmarsat C equipment to have an integral satellite navigation receiver, which ensures that accurate location information is transmitted to an international rescue coordination centre in the event of a distress alert being sent.

Inmarsat A and B Inmarsat A, an old analogue system, began operating in 1982. In July 2002 the International Marine Satellite Organization (IMSO)

announced that Inmarsat A services would be withdrawn globally on 31 December 2007.

Inmarsat B, a new digital version, is cheaper to operate, but has the disadvantage of requiring a large parabolic antenna, making it unsuitable for most cruising yachts.

Inmarsat M The 'M' stands for 'mobile', and the majority of M-units are used on land. Marine M-units usually incorporate a distress-alert button, making them suitable for use at sea by any craft that is not GMDSS-compatible (see p44). A small steerable parabolic antenna, which can be fitted to most sailboats, is required for this system.

Inmarsat Mini M Unlike other satellite systems, marine communications are the primary function of Inmarsat Mini M. This relatively small system offers good coverage in the northern hemisphere, but there are gaps in the southern hemisphere.

Below *Satellite communications linked to a GPS mean a yacht's position can be constantly monitored, even in mid-ocean.*

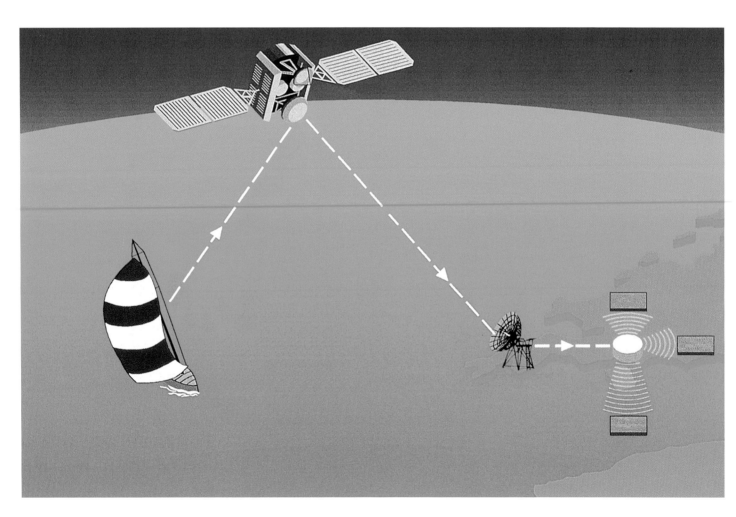

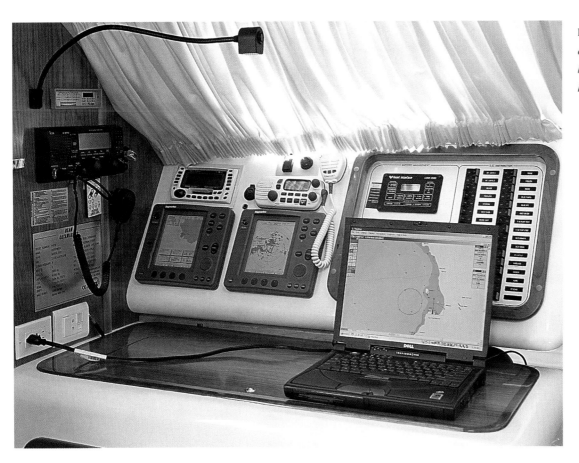

Weatherfax

Knowing what weather lies ahead is important to sailors and a weatherfax is an excellent item to have on a cruising yacht. A number of met stations around the world put out weather faxes at certain times daily. These are often done on SSB frequencies and you can usually fit a weatherfax printer to a marine SSB, or buy a stand-alone receiver-printer.

Navtex

This is an international, automated system adopted by the IMO (International Maritime Organization) for the standardized broadcast and reception of navigation warnings, weather forecasts or warnings and marine safety information. Broadcasts are normally in English on 518 kHz. Navtex receivers are small and draw little current, so they are suitable for sailboats. The receivers normally print out incoming messages and can be programmed to receive only the information you require.

Computers

Laptop computers offer a further dimension in navigation and communications. Provided you have the correct software and interfaces, data access is the same as using a modem at home or work, and your laptop will happily handle anything that involves the processing of words, numbers or graphics, including radar, GPS, autopilot, navigation instruments, Loran, Inmarsat etc.

Today, most information relating to navigation, communications and the weather can be received via the Internet or e-mail, although Internet connections can be a bit slow, depending on your location and the ISP being used.

On small craft, voice-based systems such as VHF, SSB and Navtex still use mostly traditional receivers, but on larger or more sophisticated boats, these functions are increasingly being handled by a PC or laptop. Access to a steady power supply is probably the only limitation to using computers on board.

EMERGENCY COMMUNICATION SYSTEMS

Improved satellite coverage means that few parts of the globe are not covered by at least one system able to access search and rescue systems via satellite technology. Not all of them offer two-way communications, but once activated, they all transmit your location, often to within a few hundred metres, enabling rescue services to locate you.

Activating an emergency notification system carries a responsibility, as false alerts are costly in terms of time, money and manpower but, when correctly used, they dramatically improve rescue times. While they might be expensive, in a life-threatening emergency you will be glad you paid the price to ensure your safety.

EPIRB

When it is activated, an EPIRB (emergency position indicating radio beacon) transmits a regular signal that is picked up by satellite and relayed to rescue organizations. The accuracy of the signals means that the location of a life raft or stranded yacht can be pinpointed to within a small area.

Detectable anywhere in the world, EPIRBs work by transmitting a digital identification code on the

406 MHz distress frequency and also send out a low-power homing signal on 121.5 MHz to guide search and rescue craft. (A few older systems still operate only on 121.5/243 MHz, but these are being phased out and should not be purchased.)

A Category One EPIRB can be activated manually by depressing a button, or automatically via a hydrostatic release that is triggered by water pressure at a depth of 1–3m (3–10ft). After release, it will float to the surface and begin transmitting. Category Two beacons can only be manually activated, so they must be quickly accessible in an emergency.

Each EPIRB is registered to a specific boat and identified by a unique coded signal, so it is important to ensure that your beacon is properly registered and the information is up to date. The best EPIRBs also incorporate a GPS receiver (these are termed GPIRB), which improves their accuracy even further.

Although voice communication is not possible, an EPRIB is absolutely first-class in a distress situation and it must be taken on board a life raft in the event of abandoning ship. In a non-GMDSS-equipped boat (see below), an EPIRB is an excellent addition to the safety equipment, particularly if the vessel is already equipped with a marine and/or ham SSB.

GMDSS

The Global Maritime Distress and Safety System (GMDSS) is intended to provide communications support for search and rescue operations, but implementing it globally may take some time.

The system operates on a combination of satellite fixes and shore-based radio services that enable a ship's position to be determined in an emergency. GMDSS combines the function of several systems, including alerting shore-based rescue services and providing an accurate position, sending out a locating (homing) signal for rescue craft, receiving regular safety information broadcasts and enabling ship-to-shore and ship-to-ship communications.

If a ship in trouble has not had time to send a conventional Mayday call, distress messages are initiated by transmitting coded digital signals on designated radio frequencies (including VHF channel 70, and

Below *A hand-held 406 EPIRB should be stowed where it can easily be grabbed in an emergency.*

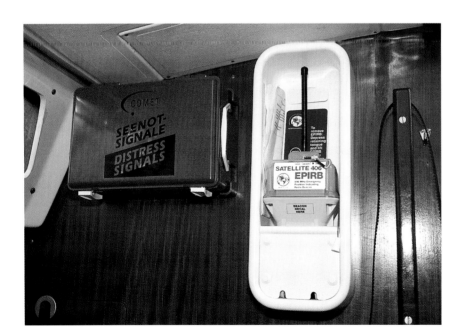

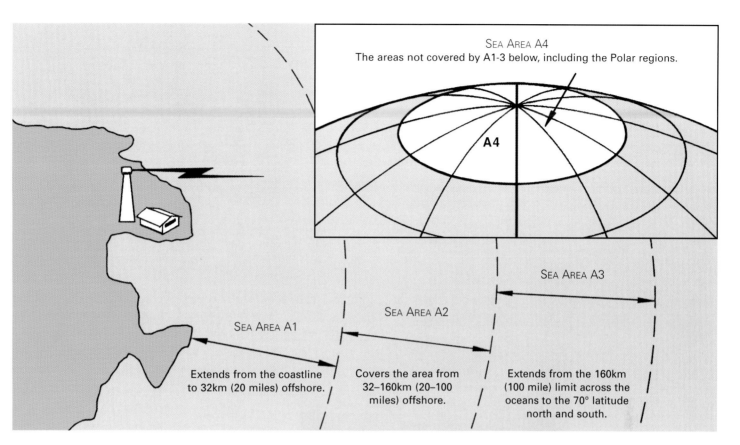

SEA AREA A4
The areas not covered by A1-3 below, including the Polar regions.

A4

SEA AREA A3

SEA AREA A2

SEA AREA A1

Extends from the coastline to 32km (20 miles) offshore.

Covers the area from 32–160km (20–100 miles) offshore.

Extends from the 160km (100 mile) limit across the oceans to the 70° latitude north and south.

2187.5, 4207.5, and 6312 kHz). These alert receiving stations and then automatically switch to a frequency where voice communications can be carried out.

A DSC (Digital Selective Calling) unit is the heart and soul of GMDSS. It is intended to eliminate the need for a continuous listening watch of voice radio channels, including VHF channel 16 and 2128 kHz, which are now used for distress, safety and calling. With DSC, when a distress call is sent on any channel, at a touch of the button, it automatically transmits the ship's unique call sign.

Changing from standard SSB and VHF has proved expensive and many small vessels (including smaller commercial ships) are not yet equipped with GMDSS. The final date for GMDSS implementation is 2005, after which the International Maritime Organization (IMO) will no longer require ships to maintain a watch on channel 16 or 2128 kHz. In the interim, assume that although commercial ships will continue to monitor the VHF and SSB emergency frequencies, they are doing so with less dedication than they used to.

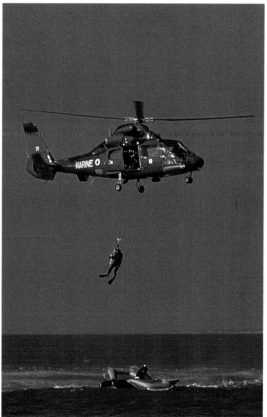

Above *When GMDSS becomes fully operational, satellites will cover every sector of the ocean, creating a comprehensive maritime communications and emergency system.*

Left *Training exercises help to prepare both rescue crews and sailors for what to do in an emergency.*

Opposite *A traditional (cardinal) compass card, with the degrees marked from 0–360.*

NAVIGATION TOOLS AND INSTRUMENTS

Despite the advances made in electronic navigation and communications systems, they can and do go wrong. Anyone familiar with the infamous Murphy will know that equipment failure inevitably occurs at the most inconvenient time. If you intend to sail in areas that are hot, wet or both, you should be able to navigate confidently without the use of electronics, as neither tropical humidity nor sea-soaked cabins are compatible with computers or electronics.

Below *A fixed compass must be 'swung', that is, corrected for any deviation errors.*

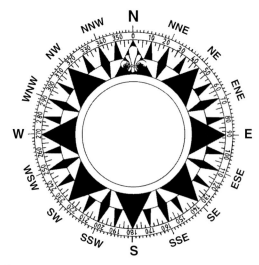

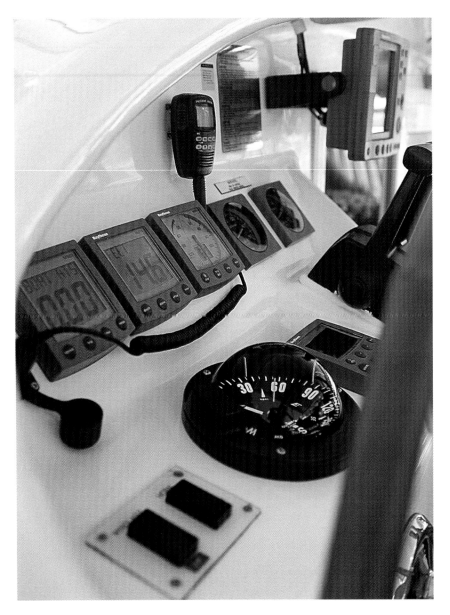

Compass

A properly installed and swung marine compass is an absolute necessity. There are two factors that cause a compass not to point due north: magnetic variation, and the deviation of the compass itself. True north is where north actually is on your chart, but due to magnetic variation, your compass never points directly at it. All bearings can be expressed in one of three ways: true, magnetic and compass. If your compass has no deviation, the latter two will be the same.

Magnetic variation This is the difference between true north and magnetic north in degrees, at any point on the earth's surface. It can be east or west of true north and will be marked on your charts, usually inside the compass roses.

Deviation Various items on a yacht are magnetic and will affect the compass. For this reason, the compass should be 'swung' and a deviation card drawn up. Most yachts have deviation errors of less than five degrees. If your compass has only a small deviation at all angles, then ignore it, as it is normally only possible to sail within about five degrees of a given course anyway. A deviation of more than five degrees should be accounted for in your navigation.

HAND-BEARING COMPASS

You also need a hand-bearing compass that can be used on deck to take bearings on fixed marks on land, or on a vessel which may be on a collision course. (Bear in mind it can also be affected by deviation.)

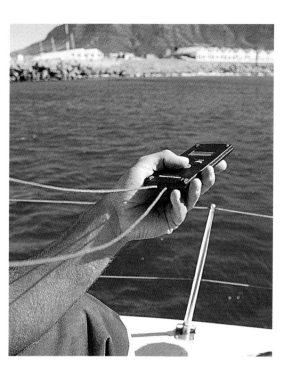

Charts

A chart is a marine map. It gives mariners useful information such as water depth, tidal and current data, buoyage and lights, and indicates prominent off-shore and on-the-water features such as the position of rock outcrops or wrecks.

You should carry charts covering the area of your intended voyage, plus charts of the adjacent areas, in case bad weather or some other eventuality makes you overshoot your destination or you wish to enter another port. Always have on board a good chart of your home port and the approaches to it.

Charts are laid out with a grid of lines of longitude, from pole to pole (north to south); and lines of latitude, running parallel to the equator (from east to west).

The projection used on charts is often Mercator, on which the scale varies from top to bottom. Therefore when measuring distances, the measurements must be taken from the side margin of the chart at the same level as the spot being measured.

Coastal navigation charts are usually drawn on a large-scale, but medium-scale charts are used to set courses, as they show a bigger picture. For example, a large-scale chart would have you following the shoreline of a bay, whereas a medium-scale chart

would enable you to plot a course across the mouth of the same bay, thus saving a number of miles.

Charts covering ocean crossings are mostly on a small scale. For example, one chart will probably cover the entire South Atlantic, another will cover the eastern portion of the North Atlantic and a third the western portion. Therefore, on an ocean crossing you may only need a few charts for the crossing itself. When you arrive at your destination however, you will need charts for that area as well as for nearby ports, in case your plans change.

Charts can be purchased from chart agents in most of the world's maritime cities, or ordered by mail from chart publishers, whose advertisements appear in most sailing and yachting magazines and journals. They are expensive, so take care of them.

UPDATING CHARTS

All charts must be regularly corrected from Notices to Mariners that are issued from time to time by the maritime authorities. Do not rely on out-of-date charts for your passage. Newly purchased charts should have the most up to date information, but most chart agents will correct older charts for you or supply the latest notifications. Local coastal radio stations also broadcast daily navigation warnings.

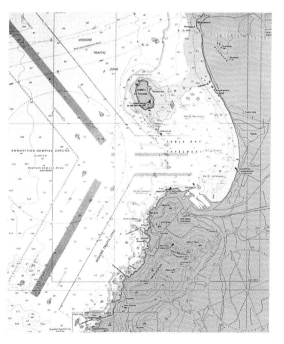

Opposite *Using a hand-held compass, you can take a fix on a land mark, or on a vessel on an apparent collision course.*

Left *A coastal navigation chart showing shipping lanes on the approach to a major port.*

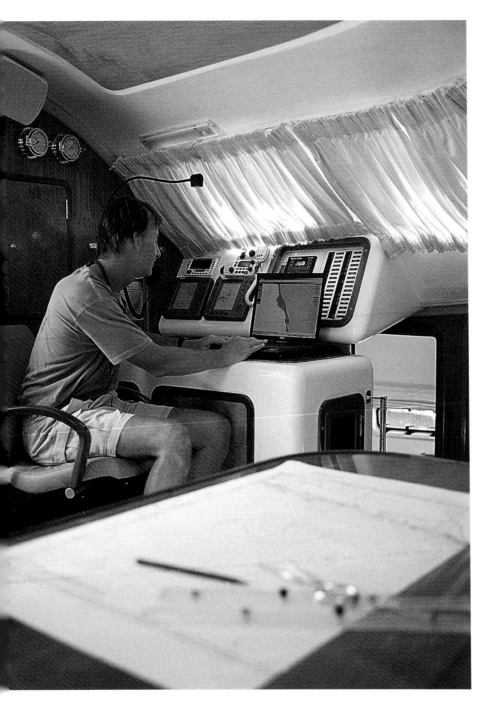

Protractor or the Portland Course Plotter. The latter comes with an excellent set of instructions, is fast and accurate and you can do a number of different plotting exercises with it.

If you don't have one of these devices, you will need a simple protractor for measuring angles. You should also have dividers, preferably the 'one hand' type, which are much easier to operate at sea.

Reference books

Essential navigation references include pilot books and a yachting tidal atlas or similar publication which gives tidal information for the areas you intend to visit. Chart agents, yacht chandlers and marine equipment stores are all sources of reference books.

Depending on the amount of space you have, other useful references include handbooks on international buoys, lights and flags, an atlas, and guidebooks to the places you intend to visit. A practical book on knots, plus some spare cord, may provide a diversion during quiet moments.

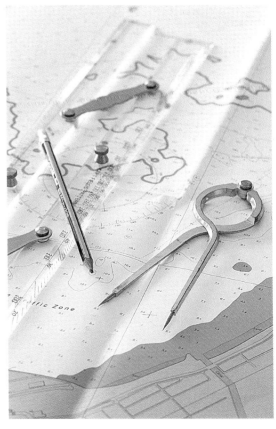

Above *When a navigation desk is compact, the saloon table is useful for reading charts.*

Opposite *Dividers and parallel rulers are the time-honoured tools of traditional navigation.*

Parallel rulers and other devices

To read your charts, you will need a set of parallel rulers for drawing accurate lines on the charts. Most boats are equipped with the traditional kind which you 'walk' across the chart, but there is also a roller type, which simply rolls across the chart. Alternative options include patent devices like the Douglas

INSTRUMENTATION

Boat instruments provide basic information about the conditions under which you are sailing. Entering regular readings into a log will provide you with a record of your voyage and, over time, may help to predict changes in the weather or interpret local conditions in a new environment. Many essential instruments are repeating, with one set in the cockpit where the helmsman can read them, and another set down below, at the navigation station.

Depth sounder

A depth, or echo, sounder indicates the amount of water under your hull. It is normally part of a set of instruments and it can be combined with your log. A simple instrument, it doesn't give much trouble, but it is invaluable when coming into shallow waters or looking for a safe anchorage. Heavy swells can easily create false readings, leading you to believe you have a wider safety margin than is the case, so take care when sailing over a reef, particularly if the swell is big. The depth sounder can also be used to follow a contour line on a chart, which is very helpful in fog when you are close inshore.

Log

The log is a device with a tiny propeller, or impeller, which operates through an aperture in the hull. It gives the boat's speed and distance run and has to be calibrated for your craft.

Barometer

While not essential for navigation, it is important to have one on board. Low (falling) barometric pressure

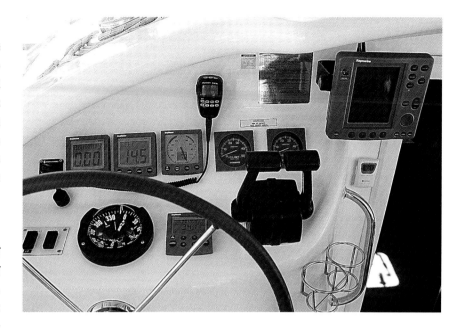

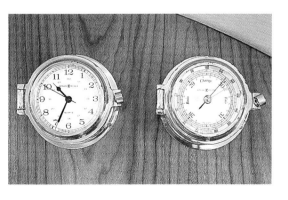

indicates that bad weather is on the way, so if you log the barometric pressure every hour you will get an indication of what is occurring.

GPS

A GPS (global positioning system) receiver is a device that displays its own latitude and longitude at any given time. GPS operates off 24 earth-orbiting satellites which transmit radio signals that can be detected by anyone with a GPS receiver.

Position is determined by readings from at least four satellites. The combined readings give a fix (a specific set of coordinates that indicate your current position). There are always enough satellites in sight for the GPS to get a fix that is accurate to about 30m (100ft). It is a good practice to log this data every hour so that if anything goes wrong, you always have a definite fix on where you were 60 minutes previously.

GPS works best for marine navigation when the latitude and longitude positions are plotted on an up-to-date chart which is compatible with GPS.

Data on older charts was probably compiled from sights and bearings taken before the advent of electronics, and may include errors, such as features placed fractions of a nautical mile out of position, sometimes more, so slavishly following GPS information could put you aground.

Above *A combined helm and deck navigation station.*

Below left *An analogue clock and a barometer are basic sailing instruments.*

Below *A small GPS being used in conjunction with a chart.*

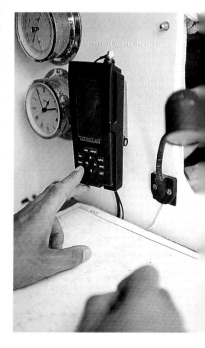

Opposite top *An electronic chart plotter can be integrated with other instruments to provide a complete navigation system on a single display.*
Opposite bottom *The image on a raster electronic display is similar to that of a paper chart.*
Below *Raster (top) and vector (bottom) displays look like paper and digital charts, respectively.*

Electronic charts

Electronic charts plot your position and will give early warning if the track you have plotted differs from the course you are sailing. When connected to a GPS and laptop computer, they give a bird's-eye view of your boat superimposed on a nautical chart, in real time. You can see your boat moving over an area and can check the course you have made from a previous port or waypoint, as well as your progress on a new route. You can also judge how far away you are from any known dangers.

A number of reputable manufacturers produce electronic charts, most of which are Nimea-compatible and also accept input from other systems. (Nimea is an international standard and all Nimea-compatible instruments connect to each other.)

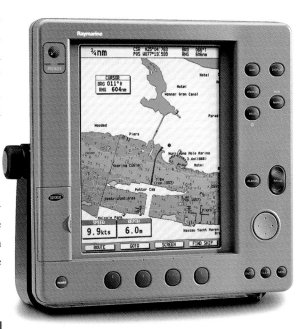

Electronic charts and plotters are great, but don't forget that computer-based systems can fail, so make sure you always have paper charts as a backup.

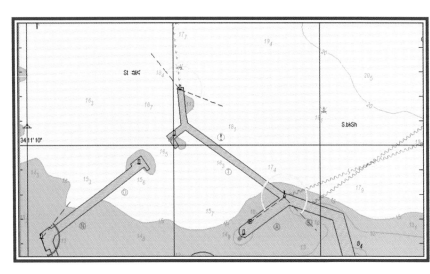

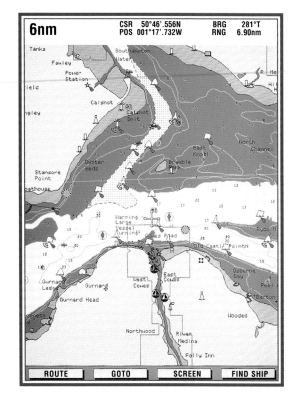

TAKING A FIX

When you are in sight of land, you can navigate by using bearings taken on fixed objects. The bearing, or fix, is then plotted on the appropriate chart, building up a picture of both the passage you have just made and the direction you should take.

Simple fix The easiest way to fix your position is by taking a bearing on two identifiable and prominent points that are marked on your chart. Plot these on your chart and, assuming you have been accurate, that is where you will be.

Three-point fix If you can get three points, at different angles, you can take three bearings. These should all meet at the same point (but never do as you can't be that accurate). Instead, they form a triangle known as a 'cocked hat' and you are somewhere within that triangle, which is usually a very small area. (See illustrations A–D.)

Running fix This can be taken when only one clear landmark is available to take a bearing. Take a bearing on this mark and plot it on your chart. You are somewhere along that line but you don't know where. After a set time, say half an hour, during which you have steered an accurate course and noted the distance run on the log, take another bearing and plot it on the chart. Take a line parallel to your first bearing and, on the course you have sailed for the past half hour, plot the distance sailed, say 3.5 nautical miles. Your position is where this line meets the second bearing. (See illustration E.)

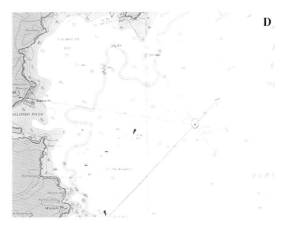

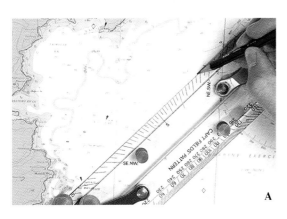

A

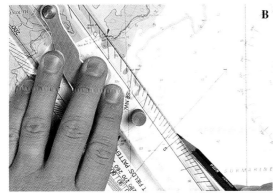

B

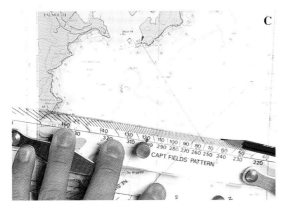

C

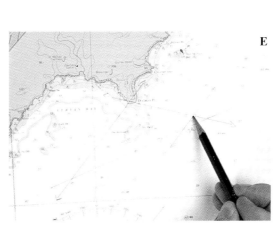

E

D

Above *A 'cocked hat' triangle is the usual result of taking a three-point fix.*

Opposite *Taking a fix:*
A–B Plotting two bearings from prominent identifiable points to obtain a simple fix.
C Plotting a third bearing to obtain a three-point fix.
D A perfect three-point fix has all three bearings meeting at a single point.

Left *A running fix can be obtained using a single prominent point.*

CELESTIAL NAVIGATION

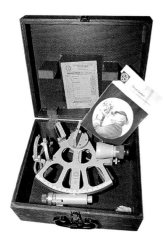

Above *A sextant has always been the traditional means of 'shooting the sun', but GPS is now taking over.*

Opposite *Using a sextant to determine your position on the open ocean.*

Ocean navigators should have a picture in their mind of the ocean they are crossing, and be able to make a landfall without GPS if necessary. Ocean charts give details of what currents to expect and where they are located. Taking account of this, dead reckoning (DR) can be maintained. If there are islands on the way, set a course to pass close to them, and a successful sighting will confirm the DR.

Many cruising sailors feared ocean (celestial) navigation because it involved using a sextant to shoot the sun, moon, stars or planets, accurately recording the time of the sight, and working out coordinates with tables and a nautical almanac. The daily progress of the boat was recorded on large-scale plotting charts by means of dead reckoning, corrected by sightings.

Once learnt, traditional navigation is not difficult, but compared with simply reading a position off a GPS, it is a bit of a chore.

Nowadays, all you need to do is enter your GPS position in the log every hour and then plot your position on the ocean chart at a set time every day. By keeping to the same time, you will be able to ascertain your day's run. Provided you have at least one hand-held GPS on board as a backup and you enter your position in the log every hour, you should not have any problems. If all fails, use dead reckoning to keep up your approximate position.

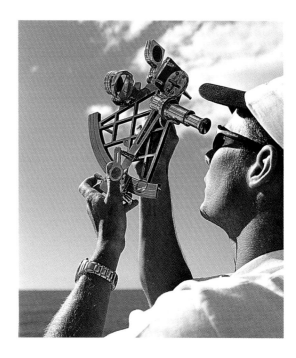

Right *The principle of the sextant: the angle of the sun above the horizon (the altitude) is found by sighting the sun and horizon through the telescope. When they are in alignment, the altitude is read off the arc.*

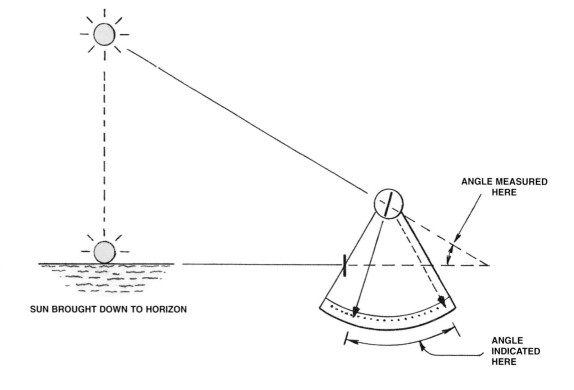

SUN BROUGHT DOWN TO HORIZON

ANGLE MEASURED HERE

ANGLE INDICATED HERE

Time zones

The world is divided into time zones covering arcs of 15 degrees of longitude. Time is measured East or West of the Greenwich meridian (0°). The prime time zone was formerly called Greenwich Mean Time, but is now known as universal time coordinated (UTC).

The first time zone extends from 7.5°E to 7.5°W, the second to 22.5°E or 22.5°W, and so on. For every 15 degrees of longitude you have to retard or advance your clocks. Heading westward, you advance your clocks by one hour when crossing a zone, eastwards you retard your clocks by one hour.

To get the time of your daily run correct, simply work on a 25-hour day if going westward and a 23-hour day if travelling eastward on days when you are due to retard or advance your clocks.

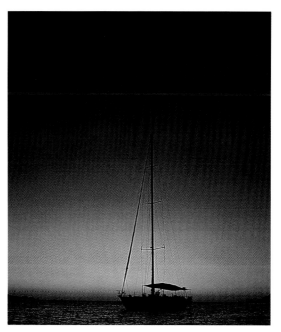

Left *Sunset in one part of the world (here off Costa Rica) means sunrise somewhere else.*

Below *The world's standard time zones are calculated from the Greenwich meridian (0°). As a general rule, time advances or retreats by one hour for every 15 degrees of longitude.*

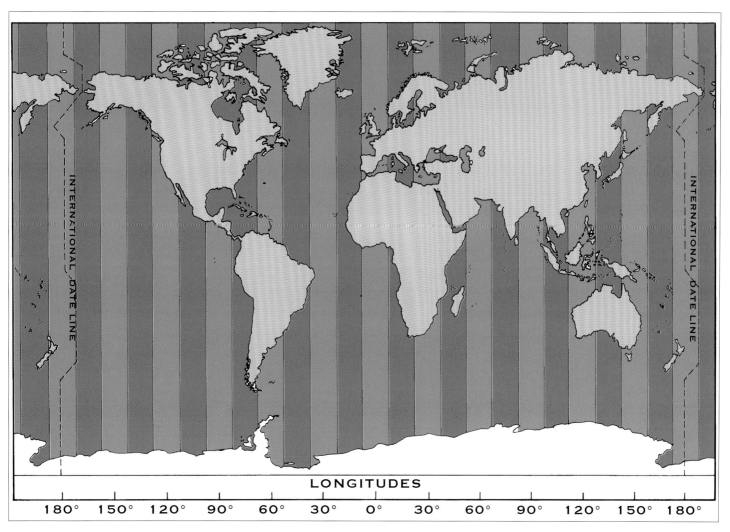

LONGITUDES

180° 150° 120° 90° 60° 30° 0° 30° 60° 90° 120° 150° 180°

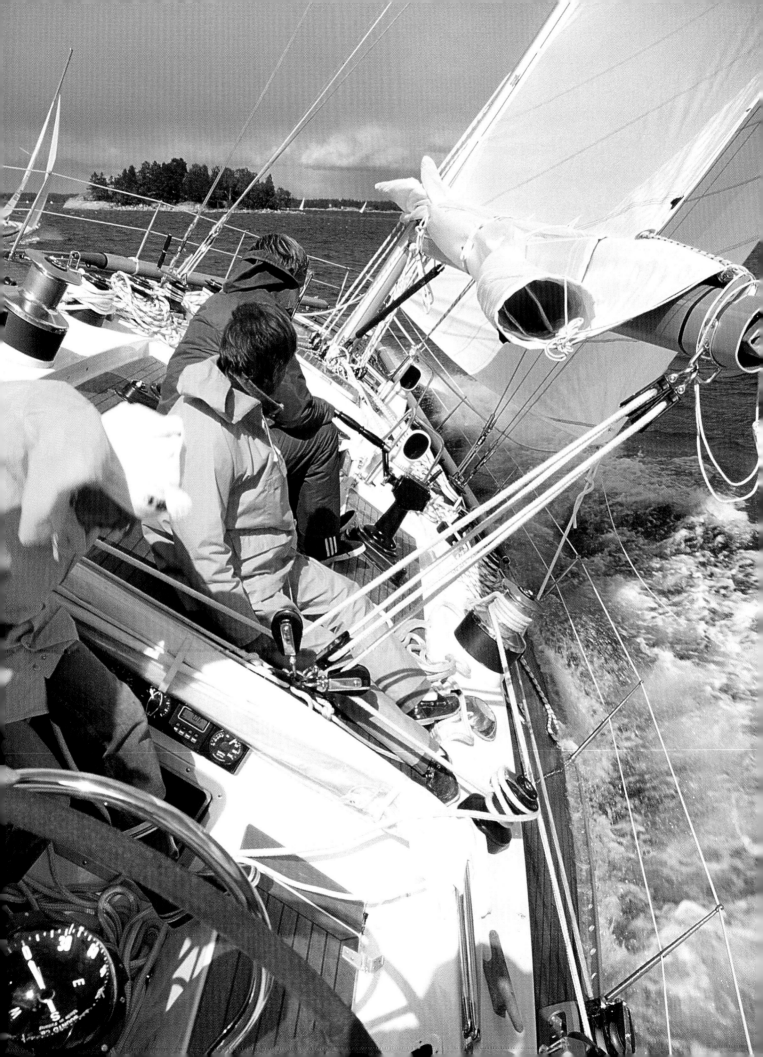

WEATHER, SAFETY AND EMERGENCIES

When contemplating a long voyage, a good understanding of the weather is essential. Don't make voyages out of season or when bad weather is forecast, and make sure you obtain a long-range forecast before you set off.

Planning and preparation plays a major part in the success of any voyage, and this applies as much to preparedness for unexpected weather as to ensuring that you have the correct equipment on board.

It is important that you can handle your boat in the event of bad weather. Can you reef efficiently, or make a quick change to a storm jib and a storm trisail? Will you be able to deploy a sea anchor or a para-anchor when the need arises?

What about emergencies? Can you cope with a fire on board. Are the fire extinguishers placed in convenient positions where they are easy to get at in the event of a galley or engine fire. Can you get an extinguisher through the forehatch in the case of a fire in the main hatch area?

Have you practised your man overboard recovery procedures and is your safety gear correctly positioned and ready for immediate use?

All these and other questions should be asked before you set out. The text will take you through some of the more obvious situations and their answers.

Opposite *Competency in heavy weather is crucial for anyone who intends to cross oceans or sail out of sight of land, but a seaworthy boat, adequate preparation and proper protective clothing cannot be overlooked.*

UNDERSTANDING WEATHER

Weather is the yachtsman's friend as well as his enemy. On fine days, sailing can be a leisurely and pleasurable experience but when the sky darkens, the wind picks up and the sea churns, you need to be sure that both you and your boat can handle what's coming.

Tides

The word 'tide' relates to the vertical movement of water. Quantities of water move over the earth's surface due to the pull of the moon (aided, in the case of spring tides, by the sun). Because the pull of the moon varies according to its position in relation to the earth and the sun, the range of some tides is greater than others. Those with the greatest range are called spring tides, those with the least, neap tides. Therefore, spring tides have a high high-tide and a low low-tide, while neaps are the reverse.

In the UK, the word 'tide' is used only in the context of a flow of water caused by the pull of the moon, whereas in the USA, 'tidal current', or 'current' is used. In the UK 'current' means a flow of water resulting from natural causes, excluding tide.

Tidal range varies markedly around the world. Some areas have only 1m (3ft) of movement, while other areas have a 3m (10ft) range. In Jersey, the tidal range is a gigantic 12m (40ft)! The greater the movement, the faster the tidal stream will flow. If you are not in a protected anchorage or marina, ascertain the state of the tide before you leave your mooring and consider whether it will affect your boat. Take into account the depth of water and how the tide will push the boat once it is clear of the dock or anchor.

Avoid tide races (tides flowing around headlands or over rocks) or tides flowing against you, which can make progress slow or impossible. (Besides, why travel at two knots, when waiting for the tide to become favourable may allow eight knots over the same ground?) Remember that a 'wind against tide' situation creates bigger waves than normal, which in certain instances can be dangerous.

EFFECT OF TIDES ON ANCHORING AND MOORING

You will usually notice the effect of tides if you leave from an anchor or a swinging mooring. Normally, on these moorings, the boat will be wind rode (facing head to wind), but if there are strong tidal streams and little wind, the boat could be facing the tide. Take tidal factors into account when you leave the mooring, as well as when you are under way.

In narrow waterways, you can usually dodge an adverse tide by keeping to one or other side of the channel, where the tidal stream will be less strong. Conversely, if the tide is favourable, stick close to the centre of the channel, bearing other traffic in mind, of course.

Remember, your boat does not have brakes. When you drop sails or stop the engine, the boat will not stop immediately. Depending on the tidal flow and the state of the wind, it will either make leeway, continue steadily downwind at a knot or two, or come to a stop facing into a headwind.

Before you drop anchor or leave your boat moored up at a dock, you must consider the wind strength and direction. If you are accustomed to berthing in a sheltered marina, you may need to practise getting away from and coming back to your dock or mooring under different conditions until you are confident of your own skills, and familiar with your boat's manoeuvrability and the effect of outside influences.

Below *High and low tides are caused by the gravitational pull of the moon and vary according to the phase of the moon.*

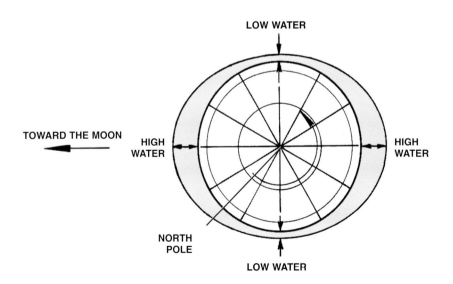

TIDAL RANGE

The state of the tide can be ascertained from tide tables or a tidal atlas. These give the times of high and low tides at specific locations, with a guide to interpreting other locations. Where there is approximately six hours between high and low water, use the rule of twelfths as a rough guide to tidal range.

RULE OF TWELFTHS

1st hour – tide rises/falls by 1/12 of the range
2nd hour – tide rises/falls by 2/12 of the range
3rd hour – tide rises/falls by 3/12 of the range
4th hour – tide rises/falls by 3/12 of the range
5th hour – tide rises/falls by 2/12 of the range
6th hour – tide rises/falls by 1/12 of the range

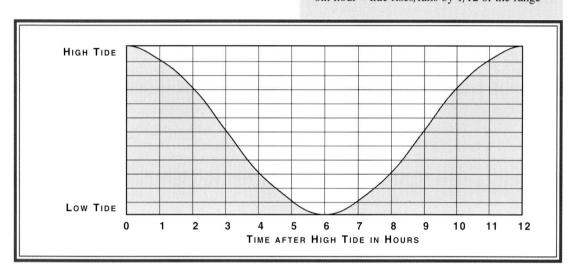

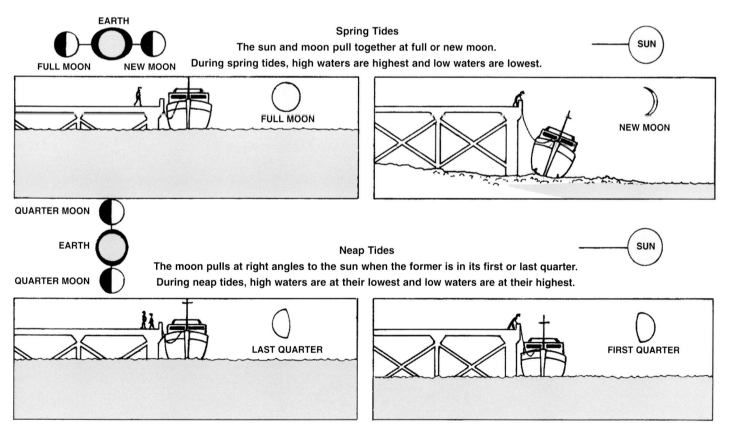

Spring Tides
The sun and moon pull together at full or new moon.
During spring tides, high waters are highest and low waters are lowest.

Neap Tides
The moon pulls at right angles to the sun when the former is in its first or last quarter.
During neap tides, high waters are at their lowest and low waters are at their highest.

Currents

Currents are more permanent than tides. They are caused by prevailing weather and winds and always flow in the same direction. (An exception is the monsoon regions, where the current may flow in one direction in summer and reverse itself in winter.)

Most currents are consistent enough to be marked on charts. In the trade wind latitudes, the currents normally flow in the general direction that the trades blow, giving a nice boost to one's daily run. In the vicinity of the equator, where the southeasterly current meets the northeasterly current, there is often a countercurrent.

Some of the world's major currents (shown below) include the warm Gulf Stream, which runs up the eastern seaboard of the USA, crosses the northern Atlantic and reaches parts of Europe, affecting the climate in many countries. Without the Gulf Stream, England would be a much colder place. The warm

Agulhas Current flows down the eastern coast of Southern Africa, while a similar warm current flows down the eastern seaboard of Australia. The cold West Wind Drift inhabits the southerly Roaring Forties and Screaming Fifties.

Familiarize yourself with the major currents, and use them to your advantage. Not all currents are benign, so it is worth getting information on currents for the area in which you intend to sail.

Off the east coast of South Africa, for instance, when big southwesterly gales meet the south-flowing Agulhas Current, the wind-against-sea effect creates giant waves which are dangerous to large shipping as well as to sailboats. Here the rule about having plenty of sea room must be ignored and the only place of safety is close to the coast.

Giant waves also occur off the southeast Australian coast when the southwest-flowing current meets the the Southerly Buster, a gale force southerly wind.

Below *When crossing oceans, you should try to use the major currents to your advantage.*

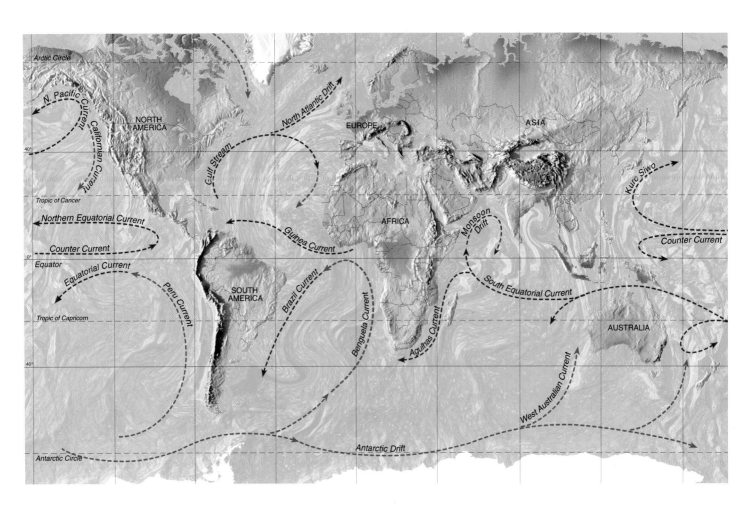

PREPARING FOR HEAVY WEATHER

Experienced sailors know the best way to tackle bad weather is to avoid it. When there are long distances between ports, with little or no possibility of shelter along the way, be extremely conscious of weather forecasts. Get a long-range forecast before you leave, and stay put if it indicates an approaching storm, even if it is some days away. Falling barometric pressure is a definite indicator that bad weather is on the way.

If, despite all your precautions, it looks like you are going to be caught out, then you should prepare in advance for heavy weather. Brief the crew as to what your strategy is and what you expect them to do. Remember, an accomplished sailor and a novice will experience a gale very differently. To the former, it may just be an unpleasant episode which will pass in due course, while a newcomer may look at the seas and think his last days have come.

Have a plan. If the gale does not exceed 40 knots, will you heave to or lie ahull if it is a headwind, or will you keep running if it is a following wind? If the wind increases to 50 knots will you deploy a sea anchor, or run downwind trailing ropes?

Can you reef easily and quickly? Slab (jiffy) reefing is an excellent system, but you need to practise in advance so that you and your crew are comfortable doing it under adverse conditions.

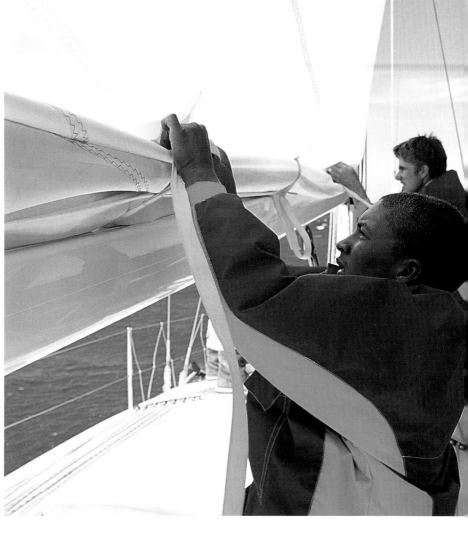

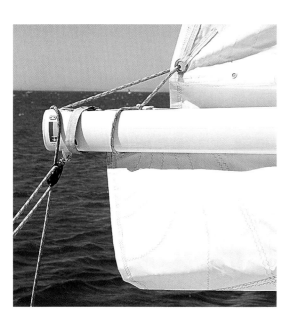

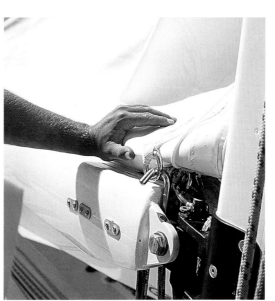

Above and left *When bad weather is on the way, prepare for it by shortening your sails, putting in reefs and making sure everything is secure.*

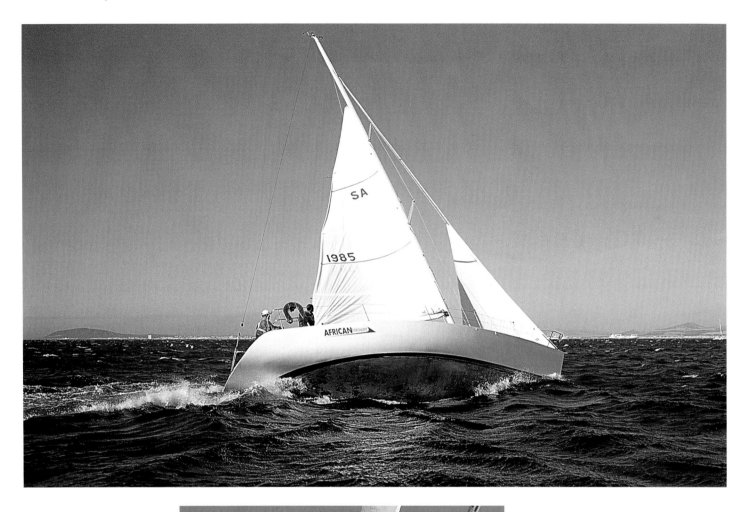

Above *If you don't have a storm jib (as depicted here), try furling your headsail to a storm jib size.*

Right *A roller furler takes the sweat out of handling the headsail.*

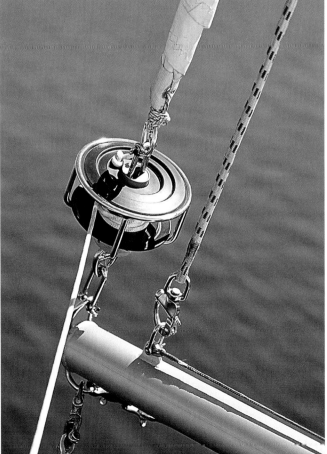

Most boats have a roller furling headsail which may furl to an effective storm jib. If it does not, or you are not happy with this system in bad weather, what are your alternatives? A detachable forestay to which you can hank a storm or heavy-weather jib is a good idea, but try the jib and its sheeting positions beforehand.

If your boat has a storm trisail, make sure you have hoisted it and sorted out any sheeting positions well before you need to use it.

Can your deck hatches be properly closed from above and below? The drop boards of the main hatch are particularly vulnerable to being lost overboard in the event of a knockdown, so they should be firmly attached by lanyards.

Part of storm preparation is to ensure you can access the life raft and get it over the side quickly and without damage (remembering to secure it to the yacht first so it can't be swept away accidentally). If you do not have a grab bag prepared, make one up and put it in a handy place, along with partly filled water jerries, already tied together. Everyone on board should be dressed for heavy weather and life jackets must be easily accessible. Make sure the crew all have harnesses that can be adjusted to fit properly and that they know how to wear them.

Make it a rule that, during a gale, no one goes on deck unless they are wearing a harness that is clipped on (attached to a secure point) before leaving the main hatch. Jackstays enable active crew members to move around the boat without the need to unclip and reclip their harnesses. Made of webbing or stainless steel wire, jackstays run the length of the boat on both the port and starboard side.

Keep the number of people on deck to a minimum, perhaps just the helmsman and one crew member. It goes without saying that in a storm, inexperienced sailors, children and pets are better off below. The quarterberths (those at the stern) are the safest, as the occupants can't be thrown too far if the boat heels strongly or suffers a knockdown.

Secure anything that could be dislodged in a roll-over, including toolboxes and batteries. Switch off the stove, close the heads seacocks and check that the bilges are dry.

Prepare something simple to eat (sandwiches are always a good bet) and fill a thermos flask with boiling water as it is great to have a hot drink when you are cold and wet in the midst of a gale. Don't count on being able to light the stove until conditions abate.

If you carry a sea anchor, drogue or para-anchor, can they be deployed easily? If you don't have them, make sure you have plenty of warp, or an anchor and chain, to tow downwind in severe conditions. Boats that are steered through bad weather often come off better than those that are left to their own devices. Multihulls, particularly, have to be steered through a gale, usually with some form of drogue being towed.

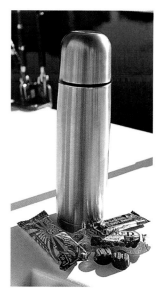

Above *Have hot drinks and energy-boosting food on hand.*

Below *Make sure the crew are adequately clothed for storm conditions.*

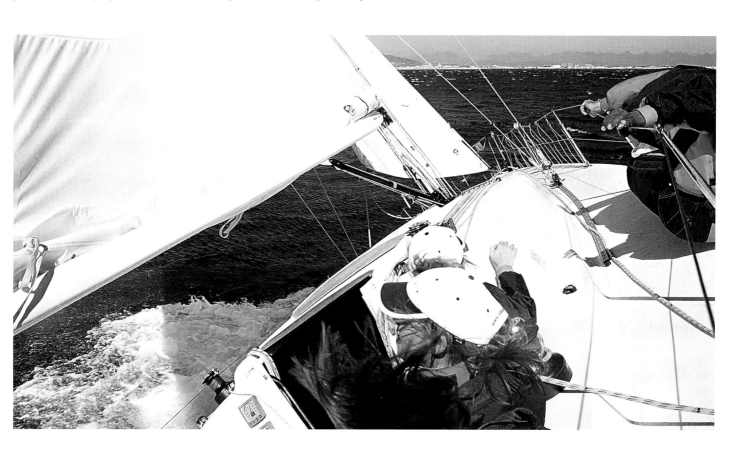

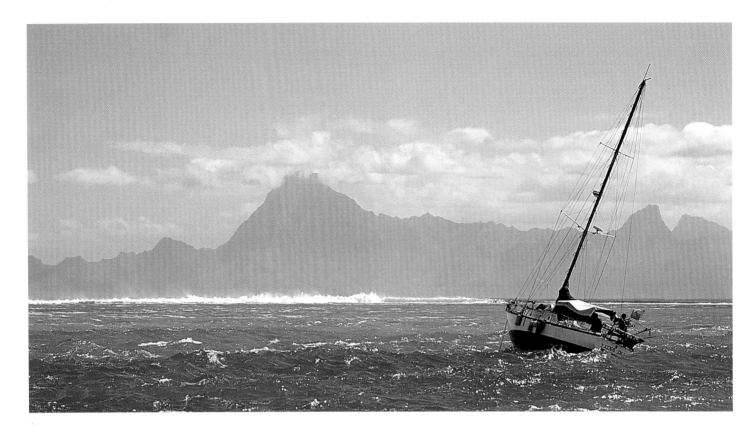

Above *Waves breaking over a reef are a sure sign that the weather is worsening.*

Storm management

There are many ways to ride out a full storm and most sailors have fixed views on how to go about it. Ultimately, you must do what works for you and your craft, as all boats have their own handling characteristics, requiring different techniques to cope with gale force winds and heavy seas.

First determine which way the gale is going. If it is in the same direction as you, then, in the early stages, run with the wind under reduced sail (for example, with a small headsail and the mainsail furled and tied down). If you are short-handed and have plenty of sea room, dropping all sail should make the boat docile and under control. You will have to gauge the optimum speed at which to travel.

If your boat is a moderate-to-light displacement type, you will probably be able to run fairly fast in safety, steering the boat to avoid breaking crests wherever possible. If the wind continues to increase, you can either run under bare poles or heave to. Multihulls are usually quite light, and will run downwind very fast under bare poles.

HEAVING TO AND LYING AHULL

If the gale is not going the way you want to travel, then you need to hold your ground by heaving to or lying ahull.

Heaving to involves using a storm trisail or triple-reefed mainsail and a storm or heavy-weather jib. Sheet the jib to windward, haul in the mainsail, lash the helm to leeward, and your boat should make slight headway while drifting to leeward.

If you feel more comfortable taking all sails down, you can lie ahull. This is accomplished by lashing the helm to leeward and letting the boat take up its natural angle to the wind, which could be anything between about 50° and 80°, depending on the type of boat.

Provided there is not a wind-against-current situation, your boat should lie ahull or hove to until about 40 knots of true wind speed. After that, the seas will probably start building and it could be dangerous to remain in this position. While it is possible to ride out gales of up to 60 knots by lying ahull, it is not a good idea, as breaking waves or an exceptionally large wave could cause you to roll or capsize.

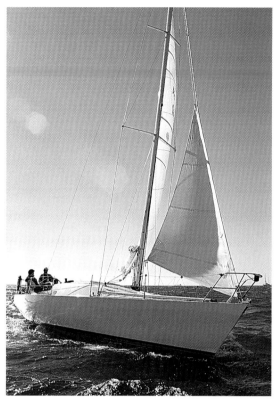

Deploying a Sea Anchor

A sea anchor, or drogue, looks like a large, tapered canvas bag. When deployed, it quietens the sea to windward and holds the bow to the wind, reducing rolling and the possibility of broaching or capsizing. Monohulls require a larger sea anchor than multihulls. Likewise, heavy-displacement boats need more resistance than light-displacement craft.

One version, a para-anchor, looks a bit like a large parachute. A para-anchor will ride some 80–120m (88–130yd) away from your craft on a stretchy nylon rode. It is easy to deploy, but to work properly, must have greater resistance in the water than the yacht to enable it to hold the bow to wind in all weather conditions. The manufacturer Para-Anchors Australia can advise on the correct size for your boat. A built-in retrieval system makes it easy to recover the para-anchor from the water and repack it.

An alternative to a sea anchor is to consider running downwind, trailing some really heavy warps.

Opposite *Heaving to, using a storm jib and reefed mainsail.*

Bottom *Lying ahull, with all sails down, is an alternative to heaving to.*

Below *Even a life-buoy has a sea anchor to slow it down.*

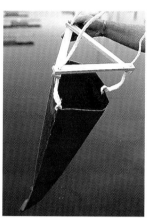

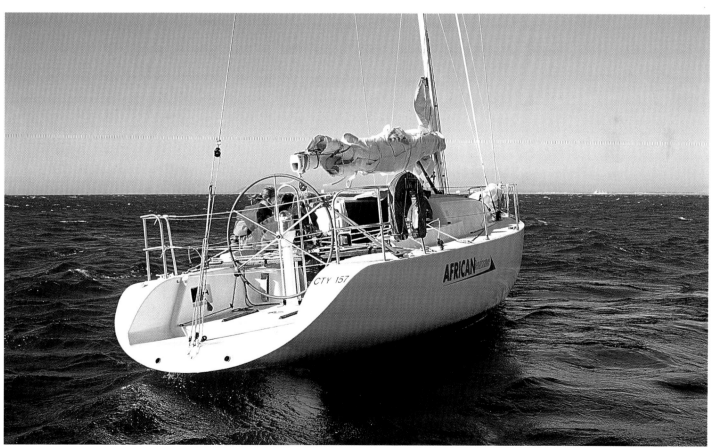

Opposite *Hurricanes follow a fairly predictable path, first moving towards the equator, then curving away from it. (The shaded areas represent the most dangerous quadrant at the time.)*

Hurricanes, cyclones and typhoons

These names all refer to the same thing: a tropical revolving storm, or TRS. Hurricanes produce the strongest winds found at sea, sustaining speeds of 200kph (125mph) or more. Hurricane-strength winds are equivalent to Force 12 on the Beaufort Scale and would probably overwhelm most small craft that are unlucky enough to encounter them.

Tropical revolving storms occur mostly between 8° and 20° north and south of the equator, during the late summer to early autumn (fall), when the sea is at its hottest. Hurricanes always start at sea, when an area of low pressure forms over a large area of water. Three conditions must be fulfilled for hurricanes to form: there must be warm sea (at least 27°C/80°F or more), moist air, and weak upper atmosphere winds combined with favourable low-level winds.

Warm, moist air is drawn into the area of low pressure. This incoming air rises. As it does so it expands and cools, creating condensation (clouds and rain) and releasing latent heat (the energy released during the transformation of a substance). Low surface pressures continue to draw in more air, beginning a cycle.

Meanwhile, as the air at the top of the storm warms up, the upper air pressure increases. The rising air flows outward from the centre and back towards the ground, forming powerful winds. The spiralling air currents create a calm central area of low pressure, called the eye, which is often clear, with no rain. In

Below *Heavy winds and driving rain surround the calm centre of a hurricane*

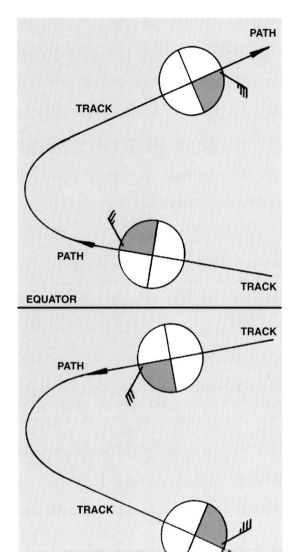

contrast, the surrounding eye wall, where the air rises, has the heaviest precipitation, maximum wind speeds and highest clouds.

Hurricanes move in a westerly direction. If the storm is far enough from the equator (at least 8° of latitude), the Coriolis force, a natural deflection caused by the earth's rotation, gradually curves the storm around the area of lowest pressure, moving it anticlockwise (counter-clockwise) and in a northwesterly direction in the northern hemisphere and clockwise in a southwesterly direction in the southern hemisphere, with the winds spiralling inward around the eye.

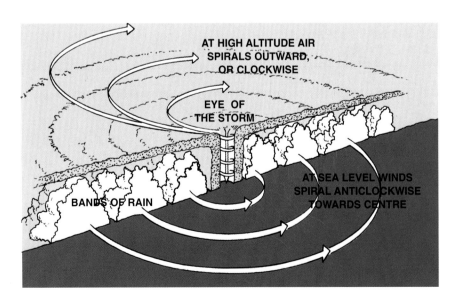

AT HIGH ALTITUDE AIR SPIRALS OUTWARD, OR CLOCKWISE

EYE OF THE STORM

BANDS OF RAIN

AT SEA LEVEL WINDS SPIRAL ANTICLOCKWISE TOWARDS CENTRE

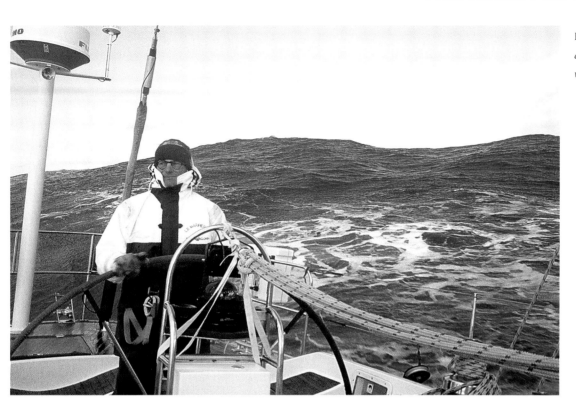

Left *Heavy seas are usually a good indicator that bad weather is on the way.*

SAILING THROUGH A HURRICANE

Most tropical revolving storms occur in the Gulf of Mexico, the Caribbean, across Central America and in the north Pacific Ocean. Avoid sailing in these areas during the hurricane season (June to November) or sail in periods when a low risk is indicated, constantly monitoring changing weather activity via radio and weatherfax reports.

As a hurricane approaches, the degree of danger varies, so it is important to know your position relative to the storm's expected path and its centre. The side of the storm nearest the equator before the storm recurves is called the navigable semicircle, because a yacht in this semicircle has a free wind to run or reach away from the centre. If the storm recurves, its path will move the centre away from the yacht.

The side of the storm away from the equator before the storm recurves is called the dangerous semicircle, because a yacht cannot escape by running or reaching off. In this sector a yacht that is hove to, running or drifting is moving towards the storm's path or into its centre. A yacht trying to move outward, away from the storm's path, will have to beat to windward in gale conditions. Even if the yacht makes progress to windward, when the storm recurves it could pass over the boat. The apparent wind will be strongest in this sector due to the forward movement of the storm.

The forward, or leading, section of the dangerous semicircle is called the dangerous quadrant. A yacht caught here is in the most dangerous position of all, as it could be blown back towards the storm's centre.

If you think you can run across the storm's path and into the navigable semicircle, this is perhaps the best thing to do. If you feel the yacht may not cross the storm's path quickly enough, the only option is to motor-sail to windward (starboard tack in the northern hemisphere, port tack in the southern hemisphere) for as long as possible. When this is no longer possible, heave to and prepare for heavy weather.

If it finally becomes necessary to run, the yacht's progress must be slowed as much as possible, so that the centre of the storm has passed before the yacht reaches the storm's centre line.

Hurricanes nearly always recurve (see diagram on p64). When they do, the dangerous semicircle becomes the one nearest the equator.

Right *Under storm conditions, waves at sea can reach enormous heights and their power can easily destroy a yacht.*

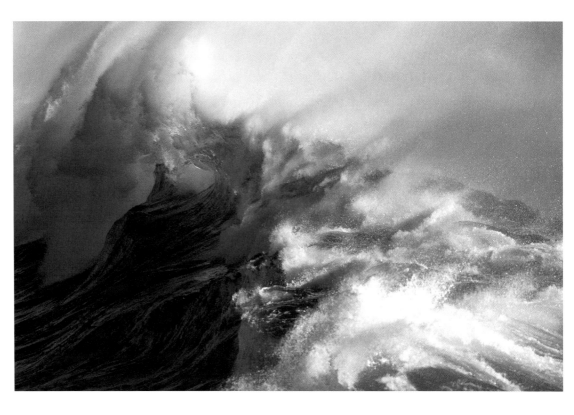

Waves

In gale force conditions, breaking waves cause the most damage and are responsible for most roll-overs. When a wave breaks, the breaking crest normally travels at between 20 and 30 knots (37–55kph; 23–35mph). A yacht caught in the breaking crest will either be carried forward at the speed of the breaker until it drops down the back of the wave, be pitch poled as it accelerates down the face, or be rolled as the mast digs in.

In the first instance, when the breaker subsides the yacht may be left with only minor damage, such as life rings swept away.

In roll-overs, most damage occurs on the leeward side, indicating that the yacht has probably fallen off the face of a breaker. The most obvious damage will be to the windows, so a good precaution is to carry plywood boards that have been pre-cut and pre-drilled to fit all your windows, which makes it easy to effect a temporary repair.

If you are unlucky enough to be rolled by a breaking wave, there will be a lot of water inside the boat. After attending to any injuries, the next most important thing is to get the water out. Buckets are often faster than pumps, so have two stout buckets available for bailing (tie lanyards to them to prevent them from being accidentally lost overboard).

You can try to avoid breaking waves by steering the boat at an angle to the crests, dragging warps or using a sea anchor.

Below *A yacht caught in a breaking wave can be pitch poled, causing much damage.*

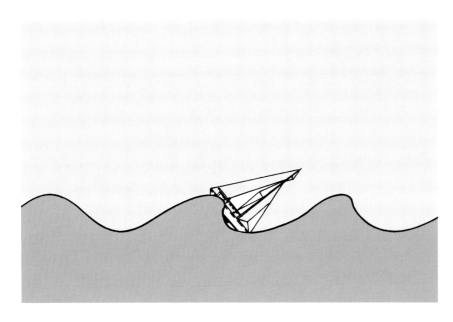

SAFETY ON BOARD

While coastal sailors may have the option of calling the sea rescue services when something goes wrong, ocean-going sailors seldom have this luxury and so must be far more self-reliant when it comes to basic safety practices. The old adage about prevention being better than cure is particularly appropriate when you are at sea, so never neglect fundamental safety rules, make sure your equipment is in working order, and brief your crew to handle any eventuality.

Fire protection and fire-fighting

Dry powder fire extinguishers are normally used in small craft. A 12m (40ft) sailboat should have at least two 1.5kg (3 lb) fire extinguishers, mounted in separate parts of the boat. Most fires or flare-ups occur in the galley, so keep a fire blanket stored nearby, as many cooking fires can be quickly smothered with a fire blanket. All fire extinguishers should be serviced annually.

Protection from burns while cooking

At sea, the cook is very vulnerable to being burnt by scalding liquids from the stove. Apart from ensuring that the stove is properly gimballed, whoever is cooking should take the precaution of always wearing an apron of nonabsorbent, heat-proof material and should use pot-holders or oven gloves when working at the stove. Treat all burns immediately by immersing them in cold water.

Essential safety gear

Many countries have organizations that specify safety equipment and this book can only offer guidelines. Familiarize yourself with the minimum requirements of your own country and where you intend to cruise. Boats must comply with the safety regulations of the country in which they are registered so although regulations differ around the world, you will not run into trouble if you have met these standards. Information on national regulations can be obtained from the Royal Yachting Association in the UK, the US Coastguard and similar organizations in other countries.

There are many manufacturers of safety gear offering a choice of ranges, from the minimum approved standards to some very sophisticated products, so shop around for what suits your pocket. You should not put to sea without the following safety items.

Harness This is used to secure crew working on deck, particularly the foredeck. Harnesses should be worn by everyone topsides whenever the weather is rough. There should be one for each crew member. The harness should have a crutch strap to secure it, as sailors have been lost at sea when their harness was pulled over their head when under load.

Jackstays fitted on both port and starboard allow anyone using a harness to move around the boat without detaching it. Safety harness attachment points should be located at hatch exits, the steering position and other crucial points.

Life jacket You must carry a life jacket for each crew member. Government-approved life jackets are compulsory in some countries. While they do the job, government-approved models are not always the most up to date, and many yachties carry the mandatory items alongside more comfortable, and technically more advanced, life jackets.

Life rings Two life rings, preferably of the horseshoe type, complete with whistle and drogue, as well as a self-igniting light, should be mounted to the stern, using quick-release clips.

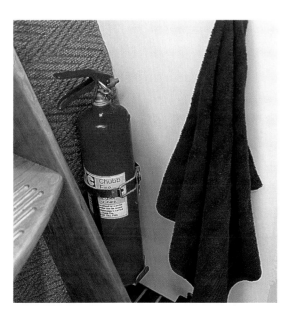

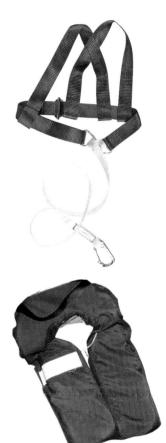

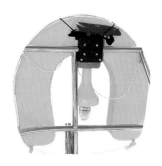

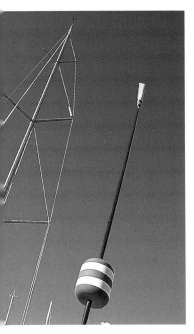

Above *A dan buoy is used to mark the position of a man overboard.*

Bottom right *A selection of emergency flares.*

Below *Some life rafts are secured on deck.*

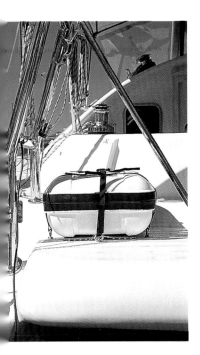

Dan buoy A floating buoy with an easily visible flag, for deploying in a man overboard situation. It is secured at the stern and must be able to be released and thrown overboard at a moment's notice.

Life raft All boats should carry a life raft capable of holding the entire crew. A life raft's designated use varies according to the conditions in which it will be used (coastal, offshore, or open oceans), as does the equipment packed with the raft.

Before a cruise, check the contents and ensure that items are still valid. Some life rafts are guaranteed for 20 years, but regard anything over 10 years old as suspect and don't hesitate to ask for it to be opened for your inspection at a life raft service station.

A life raft should be regularly serviced according to the manufacturer's instructions.

Water Without water, life is not possible, so this is a most important item. Have a few jerry cans not quite filled with fresh water (the air inside will keep them afloat) to complement your grab bag, and designate crew members to take them if you have to abandon ship. By stringing the jerry cans together with a line, they can be trailed in the water and don't have to be accommodated aboard the raft.

Grab bag If the life raft does not contain what you feel it should in the way of food, water, flares, medical equipment, etc, make up grab bags (also called abandon ship bags or ditch kits) to take with you in case you have to abandon ship.

Flares All boats should carry a minimum of six red rocket flares and six red hand-held flares for use in a distress situation, as well as four white hand-held flares to indicate your position if an oncoming vessel appears not to see you. You should also carry two smoke floats for emergency use.

The following items should also be considered as part of your general safety preparedness. A foghorn for announcing your presence in bad visibility; at least three waterproof torches, with lots of spare batteries; a selection of soft wooden bungs to seal leaking seacocks; bolt cutters in case of a dismasting; and two stout buckets complete with lanyards. A well-equipped first-aid kit, containing items suitable for the distance and duration of the voyage, is a must.

What is listed below is not 'safety' equipment as such, as it is required for the day-to-day functioning of the boat, but without these items your security and comfort level drops radically, so make sure that everything is always in good working order.

Essential navigation items include a VHF marine transceiver, 406 MHz EPIRB, and a properly installed and swung marine compass (plus a hand-bearing compass), as well as navigation lights that comply with the Colregs. A properly installed radar reflector will enable large vessels to pick up your position in bad visibility.

Galley facilities should include a working stove and sink. Your water and fuel tanks must be appropriate for the size of boat and its nature of operation. There should be at least two bilge pumps, one that can be operated from above deck and one from below.

All boats should have two main batteries with a minimum capacity of 60 amp hours each, plus spare batteries for all the hand-held electronic gear on board. (At sea, you can never have too many spare batteries.)

Finally, ensure that your boat has anchors appropriate for its size, plus the correct amount of chain and warp. Pushpit and pulpit rails and double-line guard rails with a minimum height of 600mm, should be installed around the entire boat.

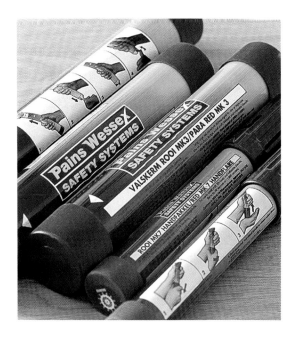

EMERGENCY PROCEDURES

While observing safety precautions can go a long way towards preventing accidents, emergency situations require a different approach. By their very nature, emergencies involve a range of emotions and, unless you keep a cool head, decisions made in the heat of the moment may have far-reaching consequences.

All survivors say the same thing: in an emergency, make a plan and stick to it. Don't change your plan unless you have a better alternative – and even then, only after weighing up all the options. Remember, survival comes first, followed by prevention of injury and only then by the recovery of equipment.

Calling an emergency

There are two levels of emergency call at sea: Mayday and Pan. A Mayday should not be called unless life is in danger. An urgency call, or one to indicate you are experiencing problems but are not yet in a Mayday situation, is preceded by the words 'Pan Pan'. Emergency calls are made on VHF channel 16 or SSB 2182 kHz, 4125 kHz, 6125 kHz, 8291 kHz, 12290 kHz or 16420 kHz, which are all dedicated to distress or safety calls.

Whether you are transmitting on VHF or SSB, a Mayday message must include concise details as to your identification, position, problem and other relevant data. For instance 'Mayday, Mayday, Mayday, this is yacht *Gimcrack*, *Gimcrack*, *Gimcrack*. Position five miles SE of Lanark Bank. I am sinking rapidly in worsening sea conditions. I have four people on board. We will take to the life raft in two hours. Over.' If it is possible, provide a GPS position.

When a Mayday is in progress, all other traffic on the distress frequency must cease until the shore station, or whoever is handling the Mayday, reports that it is over. If you hear a Mayday and are close to the position and, on ascertaining the type of craft and nature of the emergency think you can assist, then call the station handling the Mayday and tell them what you propose doing.

Bear in mind that, although English is the language of radio at sea and all ships have to be able to handle a Mayday call in English, if you are sailing in foreign waters, you may find emergency communications difficult, particularly when you are under stress.

There are other methods of calling a Mayday than via the radio. If you are sailing on the open ocean, you can have a 406 MHz EPIRB registered to your vessel, in which case the authorities will already have all your details. Once it is activated, an EPIRB will constantly put out a Mayday, together with a GPS position, until it is switched off.

If you get into trouble in sight of the coast or other boats, you can use red rockets, red hand-held flares or smoke signals, or raise the emergency flags (N over C) to indicate distress.

Once you have called a Mayday, you effectively lose control of the situation. You have asked for help and if help comes, you have to take it. This means that you may even be forced to leave your boat adrift, or have to endure costly towing expenses.

If a commercial vessel is the first to arrive at the scene of a mayday, it may claim salvage rights and with them, a heavy cost. Try to negotiate before you accept a tow line as, once the salvor's warps are on board, your vessel is out of your control. If you are certain that rescue services are on their way and will reach you in good time, you could ask the commercial vessel to stand by without rendering assistance, but that will depend on the goodwill of the master, and you may be forced to accept assistance if his was the first vessel to respond. Remember, in an emergency, it is your life that must be saved, not your money.

Unless your boat is sinking under you, you may be better off sending a Pan call, as this allows you to retain control of the situation.

It goes without saying that, before setting off on any long voyage, your boat's insurance should be fully up to date. It is worth checking what specific provisions are made to cover emergency and rescue services, as well as your rights with regard to commercial salvage operations.

Inset *A hand-held VHF radio is essential for emergency communications.*

Below *Giving an accurate position to rescuers saves valuable time in an emergency.*

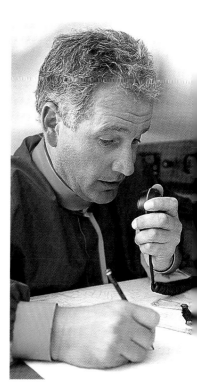

Opposite *When the MOB (man overboard button) is pressed, the navigation system registers the position of the boat.*

Below *A crew member must keep watching the person in the water. The dan buoy should be attached to the life ring by a length of rope as, in heavy seas, it is easier for the person in the water to locate the dan buoy than the life ring.*

Man overboard

It is relatively easy to retrieve someone in moderate weather. However, the really nasty incidents tend to occur in bad weather, when it can be extremely difficult to recover a person from the water. There are many different ways to go about this, depending on the circumstances.

Immediately someone falls overboard, the life ring and dan buoy must be thrown out and a crew member designated to maintain constant visual contact with the person in the water. If you have a GPS operating, make sure someone hits the MOB (man overboard) button. It will probably not be needed in calm water, but in heavy seas, when it is difficult to see someone in the swells, it can be used to take you back to the original position.

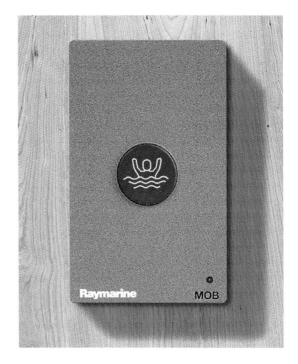

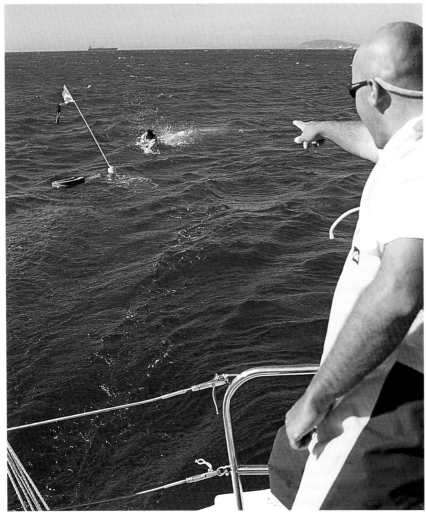

One of the main methods of recovery taught by sailing schools is to go onto a beam reach. The crew member watching the person overboard counts out the time. The boat is rapidly sorted out (spinnaker dropped, poles taken in, etc.) and prepared to tack or gybe. The boat is then immediately put onto a beam reach on the new tack. The crew member watching the person in the water counts off the time on the return log. Approach the person from leeward, luffing the boat up to a near stop in order to recover him or her over the lee side.

In moderate weather, a good manoeuvre is the quick stop procedure. The life ring and dan buoy are deployed as usual, but the helmsman stops the boat as quickly as possible, usually by luffing up. Immediately go about and approach the person overboard from the leeward side. Obviously, this is not an option if you are driving a large boat downwind at high speed.

Another thing that can be done is to start the engine and leave it running in neutral, so it is available to be used if necessary. If you have the engine on when you are picking up the person, remember to put it into neutral during the actual pick up, to prevent the risk of injury from the propeller.

Abandoning ship

You should only abandon your boat as an absolutely last resort. There are many cases of yachts being abandoned and then found afloat weeks or months later. The safest rule is to stay with your boat until the last minute, as it can take more punishment than you – or the life raft – can, and is probably less fallible.

Once the decision has been taken to abandon ship, secure the life raft to the yacht and get it over the side before you inflate it. Be careful not to inflate the raft prematurely, as it can easily be punctured by the boat's gear. Make sure the painter (the line attaching the life raft) is secure. If it comes loose while the raft is tied up astern or alongside, the entire life raft and its contents may blow away.

By this stage, you should already have designated crew members to gather the ship's papers and crew passports, and fetch the grab bag and some jerry cans of fresh water. Remember to get your position off the boat's GPS before you leave (and to take your hand-held GPS). You should already have sent a Mayday on VHF and/or SSB and, hopefully, have had a response.

Life rafts are notoriously difficult to board from the water. You and your crew should have read the life raft manual beforehand and should know the various boarding procedures.

Once in the raft, get a routine going immediately. If your Mayday was received and you are within range of a coastal rescue service, it is quite likely the first thing you will hear or see will be a rescue craft or helicopter, so make sure someone keeps a lookout.

If you are being rescued by helicopter, you will probably have to go into the water one by one to get winched up. A hand-held VHF is useful for communicating with the helicopter, as most aircraft used for sea rescues can access marine frequencies.

If you are in the life raft for some time, deploy your EPIRB. If it is a 406 MHz one and properly registered, it will inform the authorities not only of your position, but also the particulars of your craft, its registration and type. Unfortunately, the effectiveness of an EPIRB depends on where your distress situation takes place, as not all countries have the facilities to mount search and rescue operations.

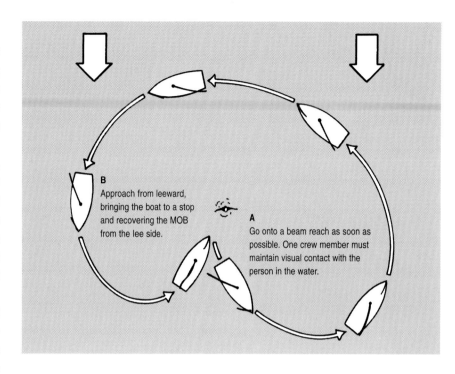

B Approach from leeward, bringing the boat to a stop and recovering the MOB from the lee side.

A Go onto a beam reach as soon as possible. One crew member must maintain visual contact with the person in the water.

On the basis that prevention is better than cure, it is a good idea for some of the crew to take a course in survival training. Courses offered by life raft service stations, nautical academies, technikons and the like provide a thorough insight into what to expect in a distress situation. Boarding life rafts, climbing up a ship's cargo net, and putting on a harness before being hoisted into a helicopter by a winch are some of the activities covered. The manufacturer or service agent for your life raft should also offer practical training, including how to board the raft from the water.

Above *This is the easiest way to recover a man overboard when under sail.*

Below *Training exercises can help to familiarize crew with the workings of the life raft and with emergency procedures.*

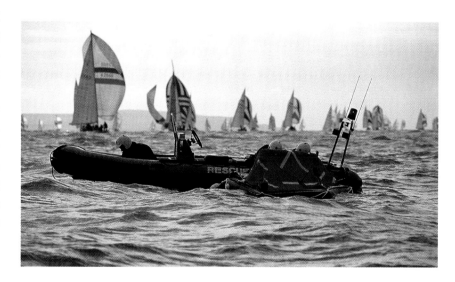

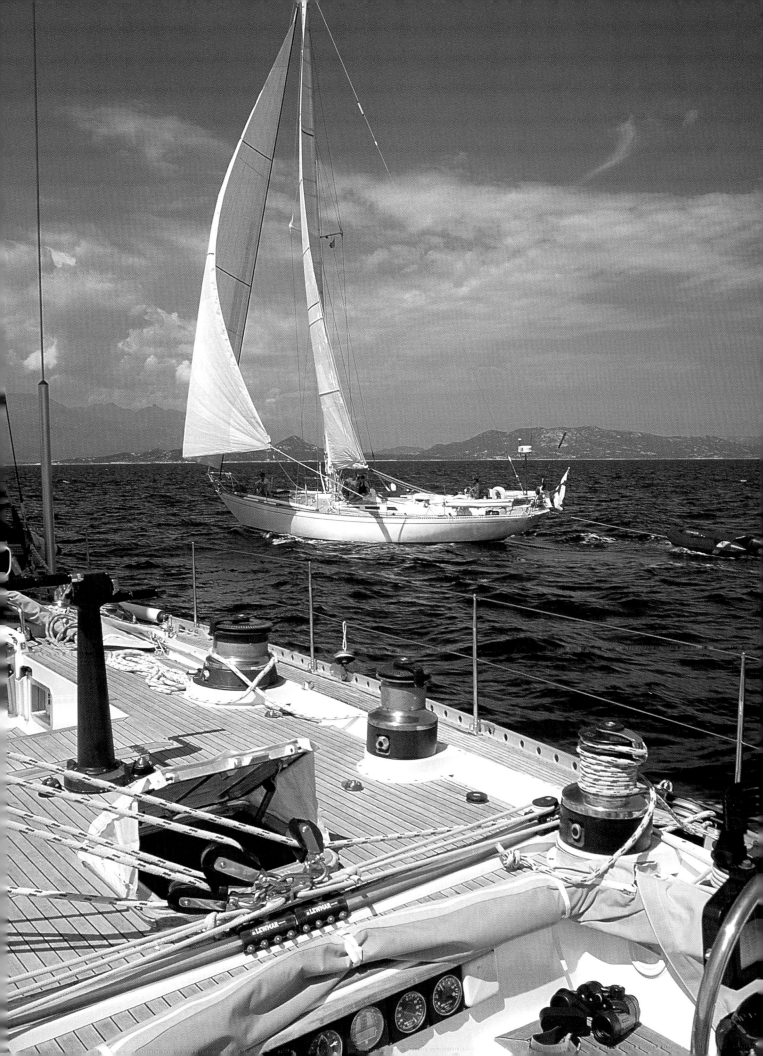

CRUISING AND SEAMANSHIP

Seamanship is a difficult word to define. A good seaman will always do things the right way. He (or she) needn't be an expert on all the aspects that make up a good skipper, but common sense will always lead to a seamanlike conclusion. This gives rise to comments such as 'He'll get there safely, he's a good seaman'.

It is important, right from the beginning, to develop this indefinable something that distinguishes a good seaman from a bad one. Yes, basic knowledge is important, and would-be skippers should be encouraged to acquire knowledge and get their qualifications, but there will always be a difference between those who have simply passed exams and those who have a touch of nautical common sense as well.

This chapter covers aspects such as crew selection – very important if you want to remain friends after a long passage; the essentials of budgeting; clearing in and out of foreign ports; provisioning and some of the many things that have to be done before you put to sea. It also gives information on the Colregs and on what lights to carry at night.

Once you have acquired the basic skills of seamanship, the world is your oyster and you should be able to sail anywhere with confidence.

Opposite *With good seamanship and a sound yacht, you have the freedom of the seas and a choice of oceans, islands and new destinations to explore.*

CHOOSING CRUISING COMPANIONS

There is no hard and fast rule in choosing crew, but try to ensure everyone will be compatible and that crew members know what is expected of them. There can be a great deal of friction on a yacht if companions don't get on. Many boats have come into port after a long voyage only to have the crew go in different directions, never to speak to each other again.

One of the keys to successful crew selection is to take along some people who have experienced a long voyage. Often, someone whose ambition is to cruise hasn't done his or her homework properly. When faced with the reality of extended periods at sea – the

Below Choose friends whose approach to life, and sailing experience, is similar to yours.

lack of space and privacy and no home comforts, plus the relentless routine – they can't cope and react by taking it out on other crew members. The skipper should explain in advance to newcomers exactly what the conditions on board will be like.

Unless you intend sailing nonstop and need to operate a watch system, the number of people on board will be limited to the number of berths. Plan your accommodation carefully, taking account of individual personalities and temperaments as well as the need for privacy.

Inexperienced crew members often have problems with bad weather until they get their sea legs. A brisk 30-knot blow can feel like a hurricane to someone

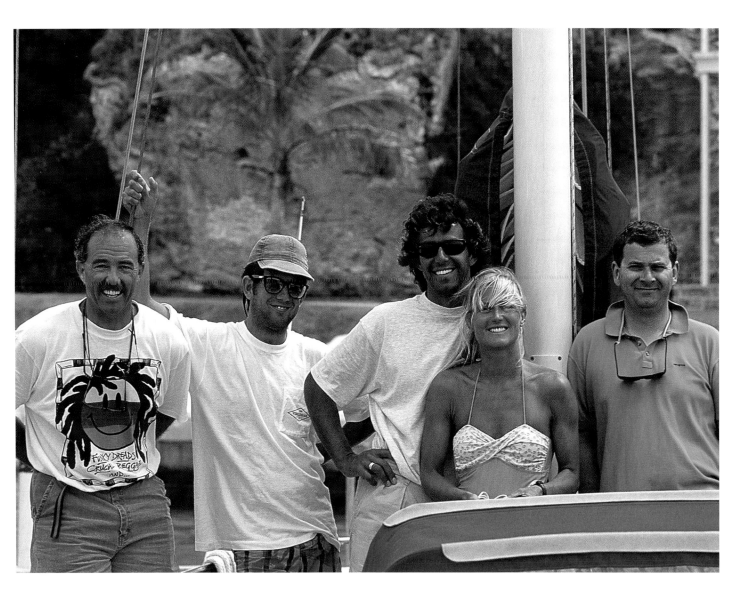

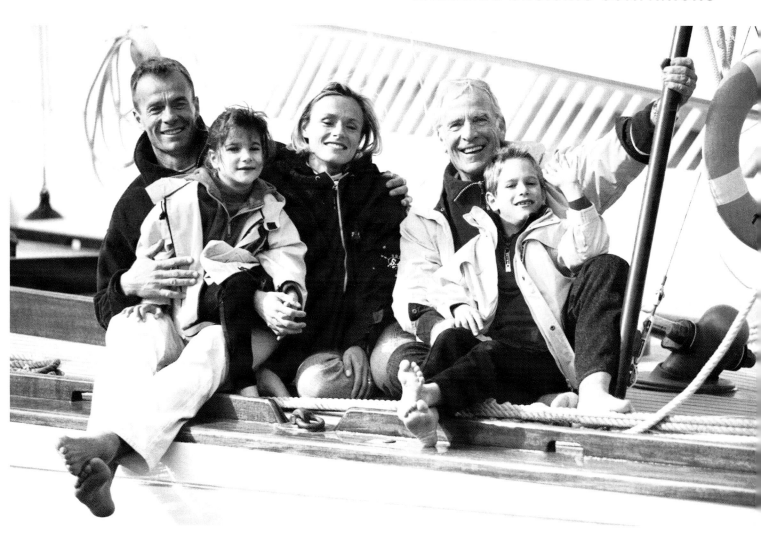

who is not used to heavy weather at sea. Reassuring them that you and other crew members have experienced such conditions before and that the boat is in no danger can often restore a novice's confidence.

Sailing with family and friends

Cruising with family or close friends can be memorable for many reasons, not all of them good. Before you set out, make sure there are no underlying tensions that need to be resolved. You will be living together for some time, and the close confines of a yacht are not the best place to resolve disputes.

Choose friends with a similar attitude and approach to life as you have. If your ideal cruise is about testing your sailing skills as you sail from port to port, you will not be happy sailing with someone

who wants to enjoy a leisurely voyage, with lots of time off to spend ashore. Your friends' sailing skills should also match yours, or you may end up doing more than your share of the work.

The matter of sharing cabins or berths can be sensitive. Tensions between 'sleeping partners' can create an unpleasant atmosphere. Couples can usually be left to work things out on their own, but someone who thrashes about endlessly, or a relentless snorer, can test a bunk-mate's patience to the limit, so be prepared to adjust the accommodation plan, even for a night or two, if tempers rise.

If your children tend to squabble and argue, you may have to accommodate them in separate cabins in order to maintain the peace, or resort to whatever parental tactic works best for you.

Above *Cruising with your family can result in a lifetime of wonderful memories.*

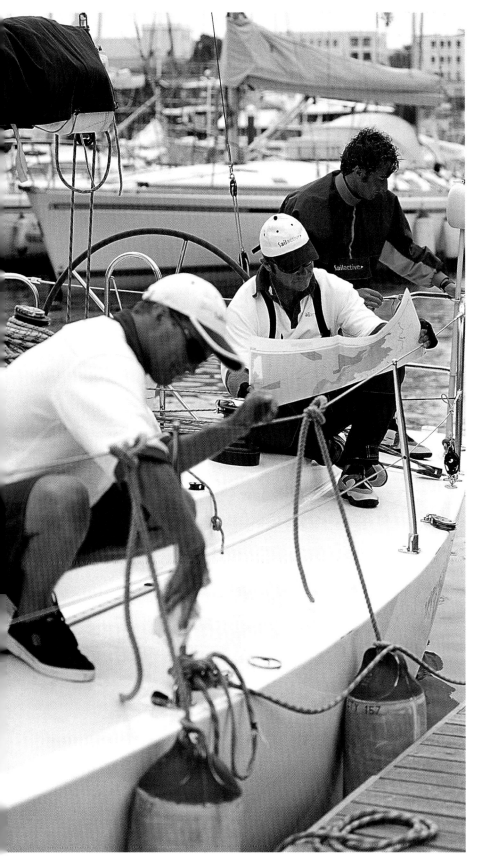

Hiring paid crew

If you are sailing with inexperienced family and friends, you might want to hire paid crew to get you to your destination safely, or to allow you to share the load of handling the boat. Sometimes it can be a good bet to take an experienced crew member to supplement your normal crew.

However, if a hired crew member has more experience than you, make it clear who is the boss. There can only be one captain, and he has to carry the responsibility for running the entire boat. A skipper need not be dictatorial or need not consult with the crew on things of major concern to the voyage – but the ultimate decision must always be his.

When it comes to seeking competent crew, many sailing school graduates are often eager to gain experience. They are a good bet, although most will want to be paid, or at least be provided with an air ticket home. Notice boards at yacht clubs or sailing schools and advertisements in yachting magazines are good sources of crew.

Of course, there are also fully crewed charters. These are normally confined to larger boats and the costs are high compared with bareboat charters. Many super yachts are offered for charter when they are not being used by their owners. On a fully chartered boat you can expect at least the services of a skipper and deck hand/cook, although the smartest vessels come with enough crew to do all the work while you relax and enjoy your holiday.

Children at sea

It is quite feasible to take children to sea, provided the right precautions are observed. Youngsters should never be on deck without a life jacket or buoyancy aid and, ideally, they should be able to swim. The sides of the boat must be completely enclosed, with sturdy netting in the spaces between the guard wires and around the pushpit and pulpit.

Once the novelty has worn off, boredom can quickly set in on long sea voyages, so stock up with plenty of books or games to keep them occupied. Take along suitable movies if your boat is equipped with a TV and video/DVD.

If you intend to cruise for months at a time, school-goers can be enrolled in a correspondence school or distance-learning programme, provided mom or dad ensures that lessons are done everyday. Remember, too, that voyaging is an experience in itself, and can teach children many of life's lessons.

Pets

Before you take dogs or other pets along, check that they will be welcome at your intended ports of call. In some places they may have to stay on board, which can cause problems. Dogs and cats may need inoculations before they are allowed into certain countries, so check with your veterinarian beforehand.

Dogs and cats soon settle down to life on board but, as with children, use netting and safety-lines to prevent a pet overboard situation.

Dogs can usually be trained to use a specific portion of the deck for their toilet, which can then be washed down with salt water, while cats are quite happy with a sandbox.

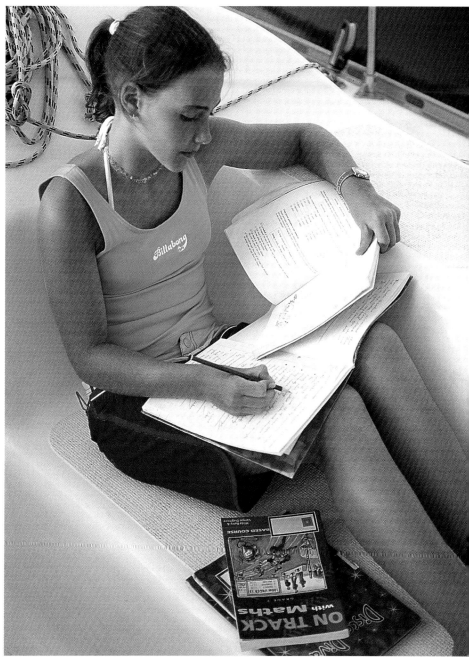

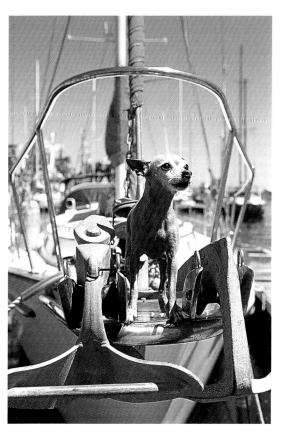

When deciding whether or not to cruise with an animal, take into account their normal exercise and dietary needs, plus the amount of space required to store dry or tinned pet food, cat litter and so on.

Remember that pets won't change their behaviour at sea, so those that make a mess, devour books or clothes, or exhibit aggressive characteristics, should be left at home.

Above *Education can be kept up by correspondence.*

Far left *Man's best friend can also be his cruising companion.*

Opposite *Paid crew will help to share the sailing workload.*

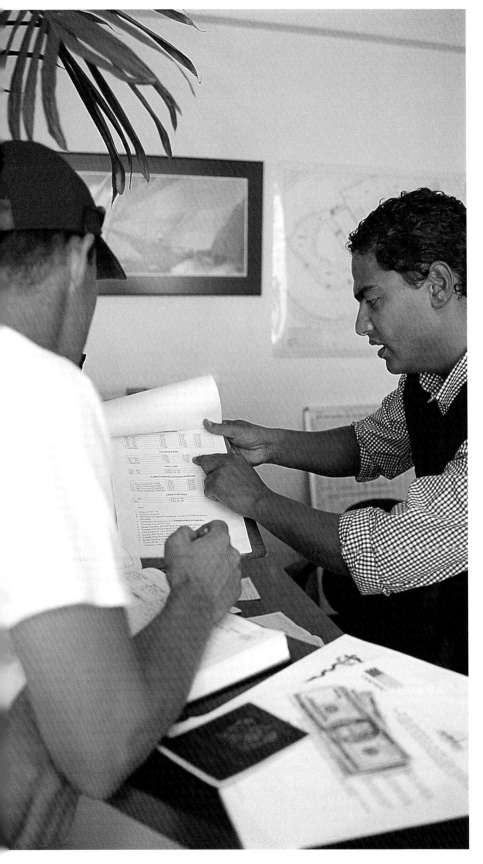

BUDGETING AND PAPERWORK

There are certain expenses that all cruising sailors must take into account, no matter how extravagant or stringent their budgets. Doing your homework will ensure that there are no unexpected surprises and that your trip doesn't end up costing far more than you intended. Likewise, ensuring that your paperwork is all in order will spare you many hours of standing in queues and battling officialdom if you have neglected to obtain that vital visa or clearance document that you need to proceed.

While you may be able to plan for most of your major expenses before you leave, be aware of the costs that soon add up while you are en route. These include purchasing fresh food and provisions, paying for meals, transport and excursions ashore, personal shopping, telephone calls, faxes and e-mail messages home, repairs to equipment, refuelling if you are motor sailing in inshore waters, and replacing gas used for cooking or heating water.

If you hire crew for specific legs of your cruise, they need to be paid, or be provided with an air ticket to get them back home.

Payment and obtaining cash en route
A bank account that is operated via an ATM (cash-dispensing machine) is invaluable to enable you to obtain cash when you are travelling. Check with your local bank that your card will work all over the world, ensure there are sufficient funds in the account to last for the duration of your voyage and simply use ATMs in the countries you visit.

Visa, Mastercard, American Express and other global credit cards can be used to draw money at ATMs provided you have a pin number. They are also accepted in shops and restaurants worldwide.

Traveller's cheques are a useful standby, so carry some with you (British pounds sterling or US dollars are best). If you are travelling in countries where cash is the preferred means of payment, take US dollars in small denominations, as they are accepted almost everywhere. (Euros might be easier to exchange in European countries.)

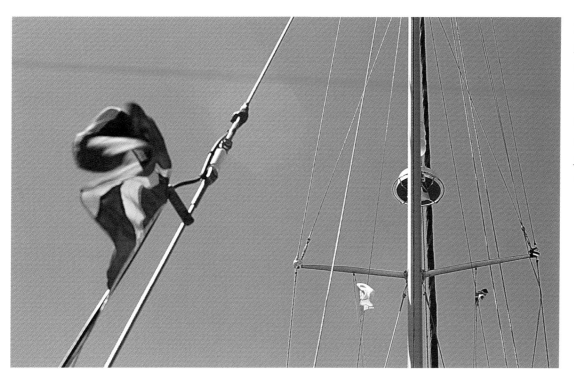

Left *When entering a port, fly your own national flag, the Q flag and the flag of the country you are entering.*

Opposite *Immigration and port authorities may request a fee for clearing you into or out of a foreign port.*

Insurance for your boat and crew

It is particularly important to have comprehensive insurance if you have sold your home and sunk all your funds into your boat, as you don't want to lose everything. Your insurance should include third party damage (in case of an accident or collision with another boat) and personal liability, as well as cover for movable items and essential equipment. Check that your policy allows you to take the boat into foreign waters and that there are no exclusions that would conflict with your sailing plan.

If you are chartering, insurance for the boat and equipment will probably be part of the charter fee, but confirm this with the agents.

Crew members should carry their own insurance for personal items such as clothing, cameras, etc.

Everyone on board must have sufficient medical insurance cover for the duration and destination(s) of the voyage. This should include everyday health needs, as well as dentistry, hospital stays and emergency assistance, including the option of evacuation or repatriation to a modern facility if necessary. In many countries medical costs can be extraordinarily high, so don't take any chances.

Customs and clearance

Don't underestimate the cost of clearing into or out of foreign ports. Customs and the port authorities will probably all want a fee. Ensure you obtain receipts, as you may be required to provide proof of payment.

Pilots for an area should list rates and the currencies and types of payment accepted. Information can also be obtained from ship chandlers, chart suppliers, articles in sailing magazines, cruising guides and directly from sailors who've recently passed that way.

Ease of clearing customs may depend on your boat's registration. For instance, vessels registered in Canada, Bermuda, the Bahamas and most UK countries of the Caribbean, are exempt from formal entry and clearance procedures for the USA provided they hold a US cruising licence, which is valid for a year.

In some French-controlled islands in the Pacific Ocean, a bond will have to be deposited, refundable when you leave the last port in the islands.

If you are going from the Atlantic to the Pacific (or vice versa), a transit of the Panama Canal is worth it, although it costs a fair amount. The alternative – a sail through the Magellan Straits and a beat around Cape Horn – is not an option for most people.

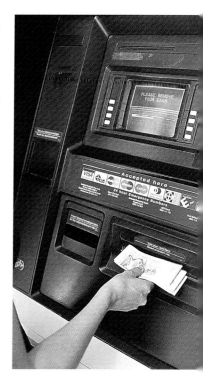

Below *Getting cash is easy if you have an ATM card linked to your bank at home.*

Right *Temporary membership usually gives access to a yacht club's office facilities.*

Opposite *When provisioning for a long cruise, always add 25 per cent more than you think you need.*

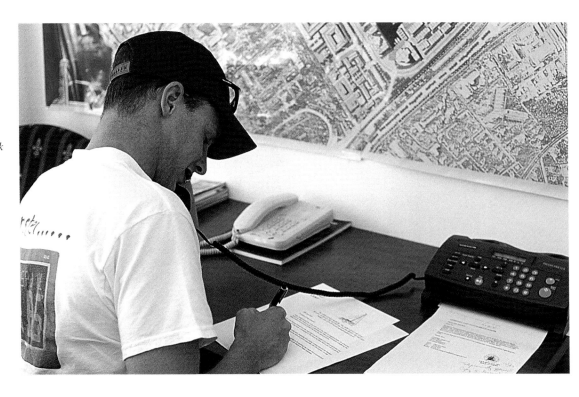

Below *This marina provides handy quayside power and water supplies.*

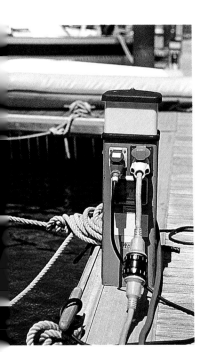

Moorings and marina fees

Almost all yacht clubs and marinas charge a mooring fee. At bigger ports, fees are often on a sliding scale with a nominal amount payable for the first month, increasing with each subsequent month in port. This benefits the short-term caller, while making long-stay visitors pay more or move on.

Moorings in busy areas may be under pressure in peak cruising season, so enquire in advance about the availability and cost of berths, particularly if you are sailing a very long, wide or deep-draught boat, which needs extra space.

Even if you choose to anchor on a swinging mooring outside the marina, there may still be charges for using club facilities such as showers, laundry and office services, or for ferries or tenders to take you to and from your boat.

Temporary membership

If you are a member of a yacht club at home, then investigate reciprocal membership at clubs you plan to visit. Present your membership card when introducing yourself to a foreign yacht club. Most will make you an honorary member for a month, after which you can usually pay for temporary or visitor's membership on a monthly basis. Remember that club membership costs are not the same as mooring fees, so budget for these items separately, otherwise you could be embarrassed later when you receive the bill.

Honorary or temporary membership will enable you to use the club's facilities, as well as provide you with a base in port. Payphones are usually available and you may also have access to office services such as fax and e-mail. Office staff will usually be able to assist you with the paperwork required by immigration and customs. This is a big help, as the relevant government offices are often located in separate buildings in different parts of town.

Temporary membership may allow you to use the club's slipping facilities, which will enable you to haul your boat to anti-foul it or do minor repairs. You will probably be able to obtain fuel and fresh water as well. Confirm all charges and methods of payment before using any facilities.

Always treat the yacht club and its members with respect and don't take anything for granted. Other cruisers will follow you and what you do and how you behave could affect the reception they receive.

PROVISIONING THE BOAT

Stocking the boat at the start of your voyage should be easy. Reprovisioning en route is a different matter altogether, as you will be shopping in unfamiliar environments, choosing from different brands or products, and have no idea of the local value of foodstuffs and groceries. However, part of the pleasure of cruising is exploring new environments, so shop as the locals do whenever you go ashore.

When provisioning for a long cruise, add 25 per cent more than you think you need, in case adverse weather forces you to spend longer at sea than you anticipated. In addition, you should always carry a stock of provisions that don't require freezing or cool storage, in case your fridge fails. Take some instant or quick-cooking foods to prepare when the weather is bad, or if you are running low on gas.

Store dry goods like rice, pasta, cereals, tea, coffee and sugar in airtight containers to prevent them absorbing moisture or spilling all over the cupboard. Decant herbs and spices into empty film canisters or small ziplock bags, which take up little space.

For liquids, choose bottles with screw tops rather than snap-on caps that could come loose – the last thing you want is cooking oil decanted all over the galley! Wherever possible, buy items in tins, paper or plastic packaging rather than glass. Apart from being safer, they weigh less.

No matter how simply you plan to live aboard, there are some basic items you should not leave home without. Toilet paper is perhaps top of the list, but don't forget garbage bags, washing-up liquid, general household cleaners and disinfectants, air freshener for the heads, pot scourers, swabs and drying-up cloths, paper towel, clingfilm and tin foil, and antibacterial liquid soap for hand washing. Unless your gas stove has an automatic ignition, don't forget matches.

Individual crew members should be responsible for their personal toiletries.

One final tip: use a waterproof marker to clearly mark the contents on the end of all tins. Paper labels can easily get wet and fall off and you don't want to open a tin of peas when you want peaches.

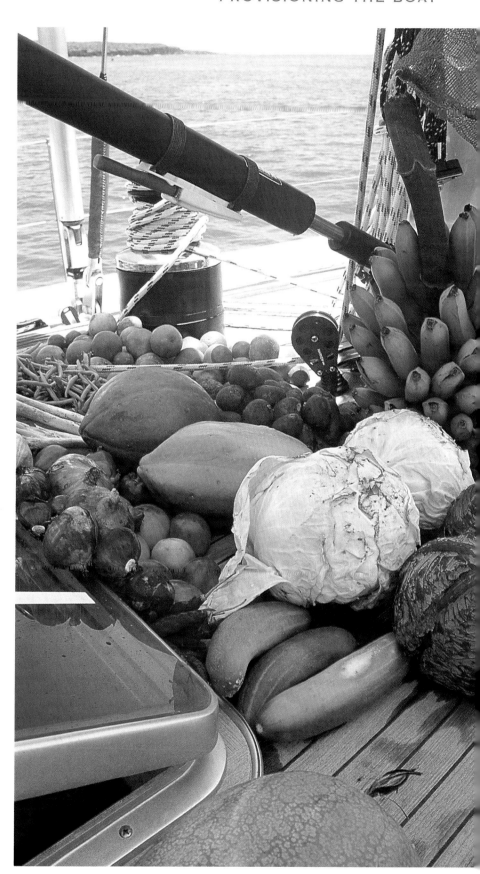

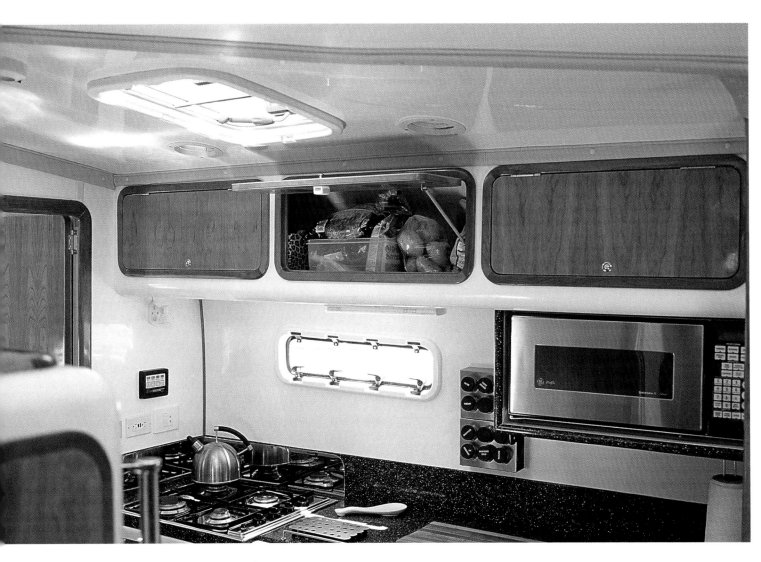

Above *This charter catamaran has a large galley, but finding space to store provisions is always a challenge on a boat.*

Menu planning

Menu planning for a group over an extended period of time can be daunting. Tackle it by preparing a list of all meals and snacks for a week, then multiply the ingredients by the required number of weeks.

By making simple variations to basic menu items (such as adjusting herbs or spices, for instance), you can come up with meals that use the minimum number of ingredients but offer maximum variety.

You may be tempted to stock up with fresh meat and produce for the first days at sea, but remember that it may take a while to find your sea-legs. Make sure you have some easy-to-prepare, fairly bland foods, as there is nothing worse than trying to cook a meal when you are feeling off-colour.

Operating without refrigeration

Even if your boat does not have electricity to run a fridge or freezer, you need not depend entirely on tinned (canned) or dehydrated foods. With some fore-thought, you can still prepare nourishing meals.

Potatoes, onions, carrots and apples keep well. Garlic and ginger are great for seasoning and also last a long time. Carry oranges, grapefruit and lemons for a steady supply of vitamin C.

Fresh eggs will keep for several months if they are dipped in boiling water for 30 seconds or covered with a film of white petroleum jelly. Vacuum-packed hard cheese, as well as bacon and other cured meats will keep reasonably well if stored on top of water tanks to keep them cool.

UHT or sterilized milk lasts for years, but take along powdered milk as a back-up. UHT custard and cream are great with tinned fruit for dessert.

Concentrated fruit juices that can be made up with water take up less space than conventional cartons.

Water for drinking and washing

In terms of provisioning, this is one of the most essential items. Your boat should have several water tanks, all separately switched, so that only one tank is in operation at any time. Make sure you have several jerry cans for use in an emergency.

Fill your water tanks to their optimum point before you leave and replenish them at every opportunity. Water from big cities is usually safe to drink and will last well, but if in doubt, add granular chlorine to the water in the tanks, in the dosage recommended by the manufacturer. You could also fit a filter to a tap in the galley, to provide untainted drinking water.

Determine your daily water allowance before you start, and make sure that all crew members are aware of how much they can use for drinking, cooking and

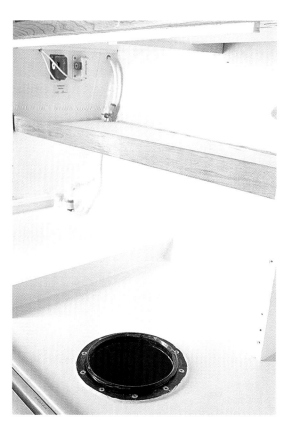

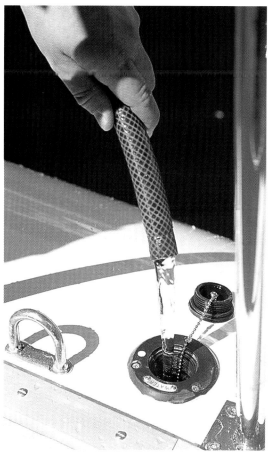

Left Replenish your water tanks whenever you get the opportunity.

Opposite Water tanks are often concealed beneath seating or bunks. In a charter boat, make sure you know where the tanks are located, in case you need to refill them during your voyage.

washing. Where water storage is limited, you should be able to get by on about three litres (5–6 pints) per person per day for drinking and cooking, with perhaps a small personal allocation every second day to be used for bathing or washing clothes.

If you are sailing in the tropics, it is important to replace water lost through perspiration. Active crew members can drink more than three litres a day, so be aware of your water consumption and ensure that you are able to get to port to top up.

Multivitamin tablets

It is a good idea to take aboard an abundant supply of multivitamin tablets. Put someone in charge of ensuring that all crew members take them regularly. If you leave it up to the individual, you can be sure that no-one will remember, and they do play an important role in boosting resistance, particularly in the close living quarters of a yacht.

SEAMANSHIP

Seamanship, or the 'rules of the road', is something every yachtsman needs to develop. Good seamanship means you will always reach your destination, and can handle almost any emergency. It embraces not only knowledge of the sea and of your boat, plus the basic skills and techniques of how to sail, but also aspects such as anchoring and how to avoid collisions at sea. This book is not about sailing technique, but certain aspects of seamanship that are particularly important for cruising are covered here.

The International Regulations for the Prevention of Collisions at Sea (IRPCS) are implemented throughout the sailing world. All skippers must have a full understanding of the regulations, and a copy should be accessible to the crew members.

Some of the key 'Colregs' and 'rules of the road' are covered below, from the perspective of how they apply to a recreational/cruising skipper.

Below *These illustrations depict some of the 'rules of the road'.*

Right of way

When two craft approach each other, one always has the right of way and one must give way. The right of way vessel is known as the stand-on vessel and the other as the give-way vessel. If two sailing craft meet, the one on the starboard tack (wind coming over the starboard side) has the right of way and the boat on port tack must give way. If both boats are on the same tack, the boat to windward must give way.

A basic right of way rule is that power gives way to sail, as a power vessel is considered to be more manoeuvrable. However, you can't expect a large ship in restricted waters to give way to a sailboat. Many harbours give commercial shipping, including tugs and harbour craft, the undisputed right of way. Always acknowledge this and make sure your intentions are clearly understood by the master or pilot of the ship.

Be aware of whether there are marked channels which large ships use inwards and outwards. If a harbour is 'one way' traffic, are there signals that indicate

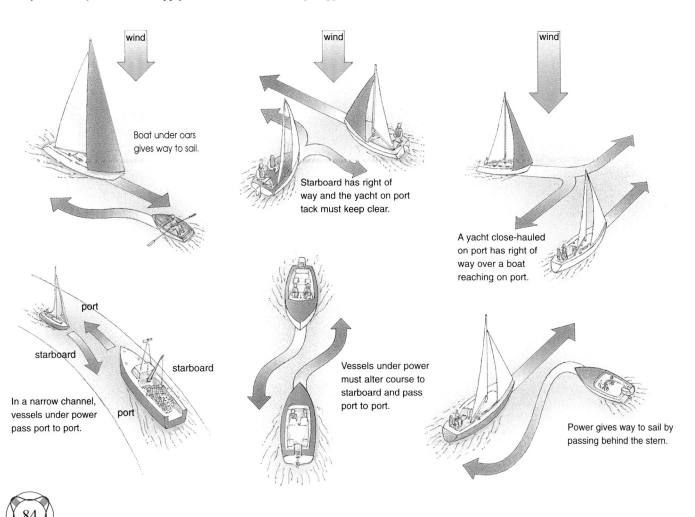

wind

Boat under oars gives way to sail.

wind

Starboard has right of way and the yacht on port tack must keep clear.

wind

A yacht close-hauled on port has right of way over a boat reaching on port.

port

starboard

starboard

port

In a narrow channel, vessels under power pass port to port.

Vessels under power must alter course to starboard and pass port to port.

Power gives way to sail by passing behind the stern.

to the sailor what is going on; is there an area where small craft are expected to wait while commercial traffic enters or exits; can one speak to the port authorities, and if so, on what frequency?

A wise move is to never expect a ship to honour the right of way rule. Even in the open ocean, rather alter your course and pass astern of a big vessel, as it is probably on autopilot and may be travelling fast. Between periods when the officer of the watch looks around or checks the radar, the ship could have travelled a considerable distance.

When two vessels under power (including sailboats under power) approach each other head on, they should both alter course to starboard and pass port to port. If two power-driven vessels are crossing, the one with the other on the starboard side must give way. In restricted channels, the basic rule is keep to the starboard side of the channel.

Overtaking

An overtaking craft, be it power or sail, must give way to the vessel being overtaken. Passing can be on either the port or starboard side, but make sure you give a wide berth, as the wash or wake made by either boat can be enough to cause both boats to go off course and may even result in a collision if one vessel passes too close to the other.

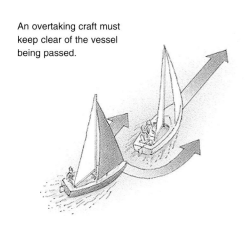

An overtaking craft must keep clear of the vessel being passed.

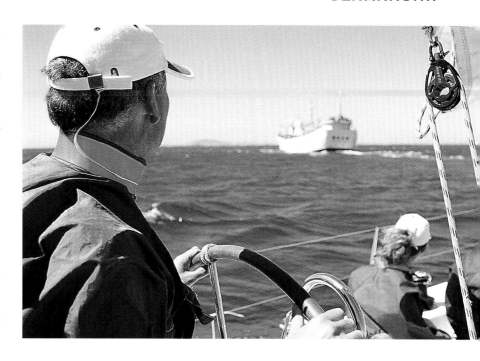

Above *Even if you have plenty of sea room, always pass astern of a large vessel under power.*

Keeping a proper lookout

Whether you are crossing oceans or making an overnight passage, you must implement a watch system after dark. Keeping watch is always important, but especially so when sailing close to land at night, as another vessel's lights can easily be misinterpreted as lights from the shore. Collision situations can develop very rapidly, so it is important that everyone on board realizes that sailing is a serious business and they all have a role to play in ensuring the boat's safety.

If you are sailing in daylight, keeping a formal watch system is less crucial, as the helmsman or a crew member can keep a lookout. It is often not possible to have a perfect all-round view when sitting at the helm, so get someone else to check your blind spots every 15 minutes or so to ensure all is clear. It is very easy for a ship to creep up on you.

In the open sea, when two craft are converging on one another, it may not be easy to determine if a risk of collision exists. Using a hand-held compass, take a bearing on the vessel. Continue to take readings and, if the bearing remains constant, there is a collision risk. A quick method is to line up a stanchion or similar object on your boat with the other vessel. If the bearing does not change relative to the stanchion, risk of collision exists.

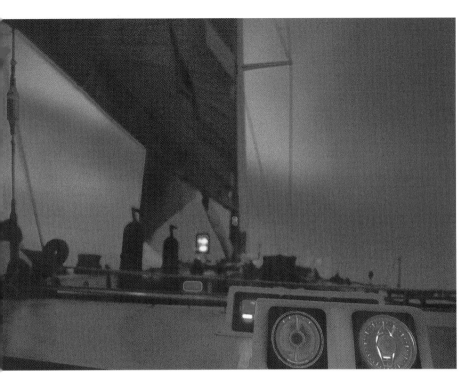

Obtaining clearance to enter a new port
Most commercial harbours house a yacht club, or at least a mooring area for small craft. Call the port authorities before entering and ask for instructions.

Your call may go something like this: 'Freeport port control, Freeport port control, this is visiting yacht *Freelance*, *Freelance*. Could I have instructions for clearing inwards please?' Hopefully they will reply with simple, clear instructions. Once you have completed the inwards clearance you can proceed to your designated berth or to the marina.

Always enter a marina slowly, so as not to push up a wake that will disturb other craft, and also so that you are ready for anything unexpected. Obey the rule of the road and enter on the starboard side. Have your fenders tied in position and laid out on the deck, ready to push over in an instant, and your dock lines in place so you are ready when a berth is indicated to you or you arrive at the visitor's berth.

Above *Illuminated deck instruments are essential for night watches.*

Opposite *Have fenders in place and mooring lines ready when entering a marina.*

If you are making a long passage and would like to set watches, there are many systems that can be followed. If your crew is small, you may have to operate a watch-on-watch system – simply put, you are either on watch or off. Bigger crews mean that you can have a system where you do every third watch.

A good system is two six-hour watches during the day and three four-hour watches through the night. This automatically 'dogs' the watches – it ensures that if you have the sunset watch one day, you won't have it again the next. A typical watch schedule looks like this: 06h00 to 12h00; 12h00 to 18h00; 18h00 to 22h00; 22h00 to 02h00; 02h00 to 06h00.

Unless you have a dedicated cook, change watch times to coincide with meals, so eating is done at the start of a watch. Generally, the watch going off duty does the cooking and all the crew eat together, then the watch coming on duty does the washing up. (A word about washing up, which no-one is keen on. It must be done immediately after a meal, preferably not by the person who cooked. That way, everything will be ready for the next cook, and galley duty won't be such a chore!)

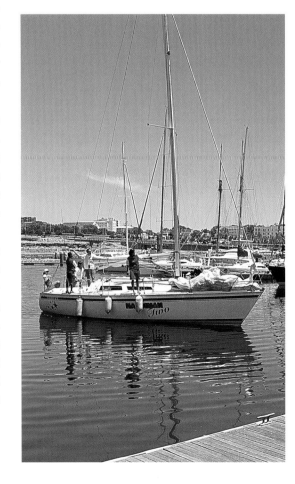

NONVERBAL COMMUNICATIONS – LIGHTS, SOUND, BUOYS, FLAGS

Navigation lights

Because the configuration of navigation lights is spelt out in the international Colregs, by looking at a vessel's navigation lights at night, you can tell what it is and, most importantly, which way it is going.

The absence of white steaming lights indicates that a vessel is being driven by sail. All sailboat navigation lights should meet the minimum levels of visibility specified in the Colregs. Yachts are permitted several combinations of lights, all of which are legal.

A vessel under sail must display both a port and a starboard light, which can be housed in one lantern, and a stern light. These can all be combined in what is known as a tricolour, mounted at the masthead. This is an economical option as it only uses one bulb. It is also highly visible at sea where there are no background lights. The tricolour is a sailing light only and must be switched off as soon as you start your engine. (Although the tricolour is an excellent light at sea, it should not be used in harbours as it easily merges with the background lights, while the sailboat's hull remains invisible in the darkness.)

When you are under power, the lower port, starboard and stern lights must be switched on together with a white steaming light, mounted at least 2m (6½ft) higher than the others. A steaming light switched on together with a tricolour is wrong, and makes things difficult for commercial pilots.

The angles through which the lights must shine are clearly defined in the Colregs. When just aft of the beam, the port, starboard and steaming lights will cease to be visible. The vessel will then show a single stern light.

IDENTIFYING OTHER VESSELS BY THEIR LIGHTS

Fishing boats such as stern trawlers, long-line vessels, drift-net trawlers and others can be identified by day by their specific shapes and at night by their lights. Working boats can carry out completely unexpected manoeuvres and are best given a wide margin.

NAVIGATION LIGHTS

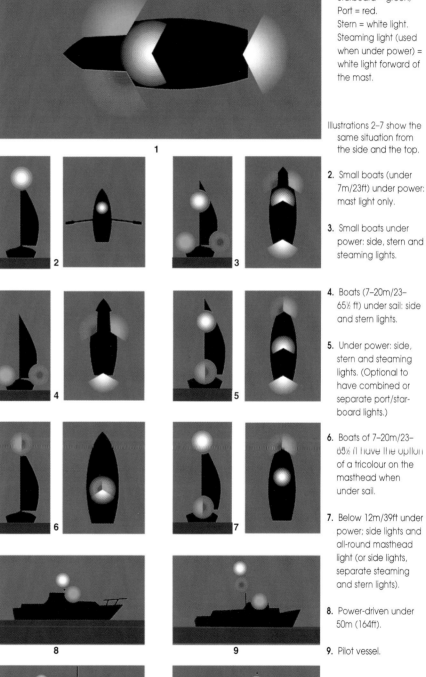

1. Side lights: Starboard = green; Port = red. Stern = white light. Steaming light (used when under power) = white light forward of the mast.

Illustrations 2–7 show the same situation from the side and the top.

2. Small boats (under 7m/23ft) under power: mast light only.

3. Small boats under power: side, stern and steaming lights.

4. Boats (7–20m/23–65½ ft) under sail: side and stern lights.

5. Under power: side, stern and steaming lights. (Optional to have combined or separate port/starboard lights.)

6. Boats of 7–20m/23–65½ ft have the option of a tricolour on the masthead when under sail.

7. Below 12m/39ft under power; side lights and all-round masthead light (or side lights, separate steaming and stern lights).

8. Power-driven under 50m (164ft).

9. Pilot vessel.

10. Power-driven vessel over 50m (164ft).

11. At anchor (all-round white light).

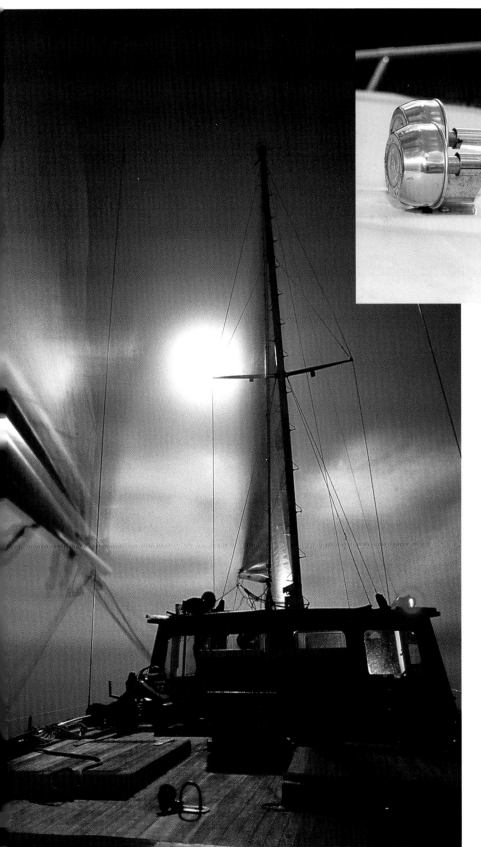

Sound signals

One short blast on a ship's whistle means it is turning to starboard, two short blasts signal a turn to port, and three short blasts mean the engines are running astern.

Five short blasts indicate 'get out of the way' and are often given by a commercial vessel entering an area where there is heavy leisure-craft activity. The same signal may be directed at a boat whose intentions are not clear, but which is obliged to give way.

In a narrow channel, if a vessel coming up astern gives two long blasts followed by a short one, it intends to overtake on the starboard side. Two long blasts and two short in the same situation means it intends to overtake to port. Sailboats are not expected to answer, but if you choose to do so, four blasts (one long, one short, one long, one short) mean 'I understand and will hold my course'.

Top *An air horn is used to make sound signals.*

Left *After dark, navigation lights must be clearly visible.*

Buoys

Although buoyage systems vary around the world, most countries comply with IALA (International Association of Lighthouse Authorities) recommendations. Buoyage is always mentioned in pilots, and buoys and their characteristics are marked on large-scale charts, so do your homework before you arrive in strange waters.

All European waters, and most of the rest of the world (with the exception of the USA and some Pacific Rim countries) operate the IALA System-A buoyage. The basics of this system are that on entering a port or river, the port-side marks are red (and flash red at night), while the starboard marks are green (and flash green at night).

Marks or buoys that mark channels, rivers and ports are called lateral buoys, while cardinal marks indicate the north, south, east and west side of dangers. Other marks which should be kept in mind are isolated danger marks, safe water and special marks.

Remember that the USA, Japan and the Philippines all operate on the IALA System-B, which is the reverse of System-A.

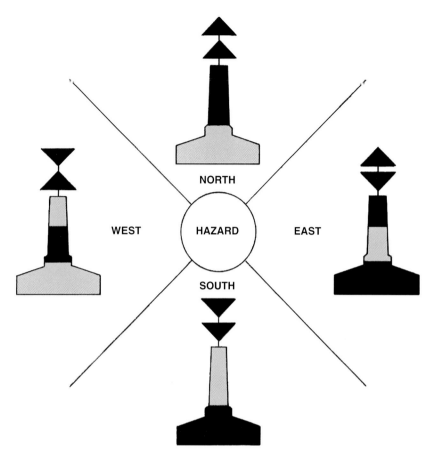

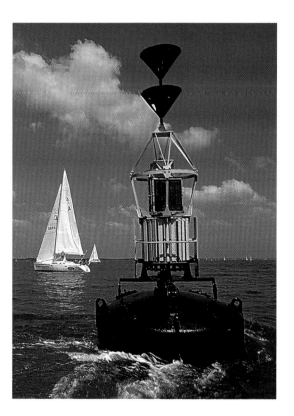

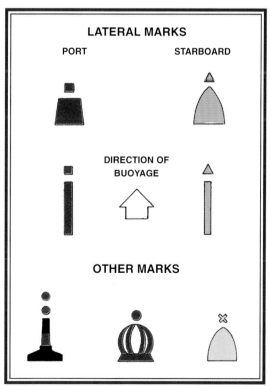

Above *The Cardinal System uses yellow (or white) and black buoys to indicate hazards. The specific colour pattern, top marks and light characteristics of each buoy helps a navigator to determine the exact compass quadrant of the hazard when viewed from the buoy.*

Left *The lateral marks of IALA System-A indicate channels as seen when approaching from seaward.*

Opposite *This buoy marks a danger or hazard lying to the north of it.*

Flags

Although flags are no longer used for signalling or sending messages, there are certain traditions that should be observed by visiting yachts.

Fly your own national flag (or that of the country in which your boat is registered) from the stern of your craft, using a short flagpole or the backstay.

While you are in a foreign country, fly their flag from your starboard spreader. If you are unable to obtain the proper flag before you leave home, try and obtain one en route, or purchase a national flag as soon as possible after your arrival in a new country.

Use a short flagpole or the backstay to fly your national flag from the stern.

Some foreign ports have been known to fine visitors for not flying a courtesy flag when visiting their country. (Brazil is one, an important factor for entrants in the Cape to Rio Race!)

It is customary to fly the Q flag (a yellow flag) from the starboard spreader when first entering a port in a different country. The Q flag indicates that everybody on board is in good health and you would like to be cleared by the port health authorities.

When making a lengthy voyage, always carry some spare national flags, as it is very unseamanlike to have a tatty flag flying from your stern.

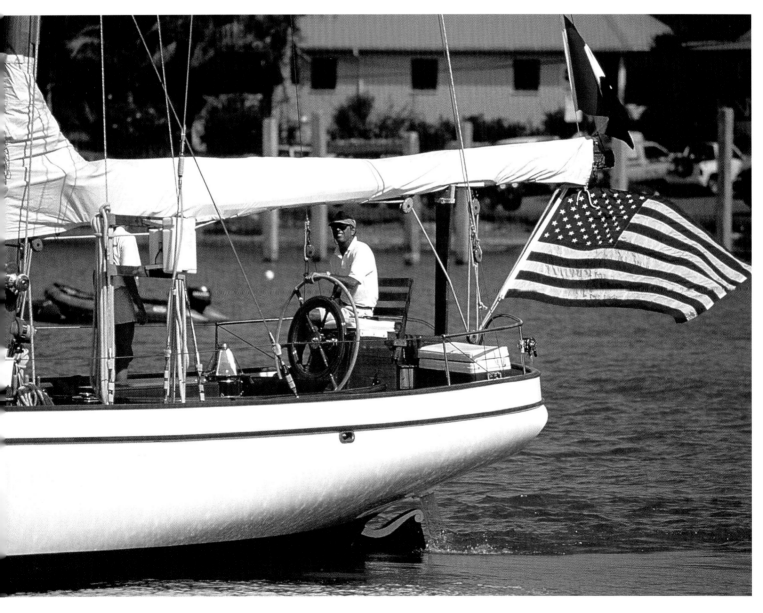

INTERNATIONAL FLAG CODE SYSTEM

A · B · C · D · FS

E · F · G · H · SS

· TS

I · J · K · L · 1

M · N · O · P · 2

· 3

Q · R · S · T · 4

· 5

· 6

U · V · W · X · 7

· 8

Y · Z · AP + CF · 0 (zero) · 9

A (Alpha)	I have a diver down; keep clear and pass at low speed.
B (Bravo)	I am loading, unloading or carrying dangerous goods.
C (Charlie)	Yes; confirmation of preceding signal.
D (Delta)	Keep clear, I am manoeuvring with difficulty.
E (Echo)	I am altering course to starboard.
F (Foxtrot)	I am disabled, communicate with me.
G (Golf)	I require a pilot or (on fishing vessel) I am hauling in nets.
H (Hotel)	I have a pilot on board.
I (India)	I am altering course to port.
J (Juliet)	I am on fire and have dangerous cargo on board; keep clear.
K (Kilo)	I wish to communicate with you.
L (Lima)	You should stop your vessel immediately.
M (Mike)	My vessel is stopped and making no way through the water.
N (November)	No; the preceding signal should be read in the negative.
O (Oscar)	Man overboard.
P (Papa)	I am about to put to sea.
Q (Quebec)	My vessel is healthy and I request clearance to come ashore.
R (Romeo)	Single letter code R has no allocated meaning; see the IRPCS.
S (Sierra)	I am going astern under power.
T (Tango)	Keep clear, I am engaged in pair trawling.
U (Uniform)	You are running into danger.
V (Victor)	I require assistance.
W (Whisky)	I require medical assistance.
X (X-ray)	Stop carrying out your intentions and watch for my signals.
Y (Yankee)	I am dragging my anchor.
Z (Zulu)	I require a tug or (on a fishing vessel) I am shooting nets.
AP + CF	Answering pennant and code flag. The code flag is flown to show that the International Code is being used, and to acknowledge a message.
FS	First substitute.
SS	Second substitute.
TS	Third substitute.
0 (zero) to 9	Numerals.

KNOTS

This book assumes you are not a novice sailor and can therefore tie the necessary knots. The following are the most important knots a sailor needs to know.

Bowline A most useful knot for mooring, tying sheets to a sail and any number of other tasks. It can be undone under load.

Reef (Square) Knot Used, as its name implies, for tying down a reef. Can be undone under load.

Figure of Eight Usually used for a stop knot at the end of sheets to prevent them being lost by going through a block or lead.

Round Turn and Two Half-hitches Used on mooring lines and to tie a rope to a fixed point.

Clove Hitch For tying a rope to a spar or post.

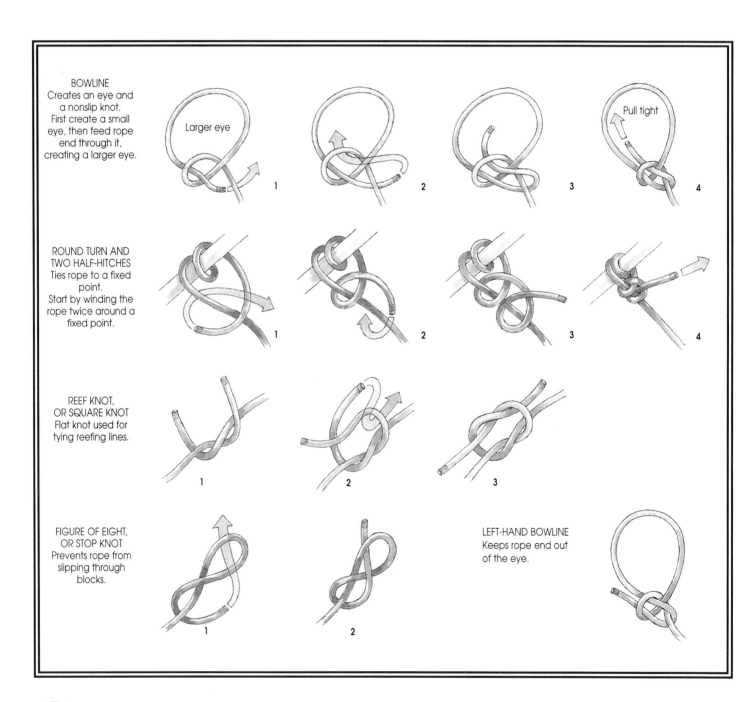

BOWLINE
Creates an eye and a nonslip knot.
First create a small eye, then feed rope end through it, creating a larger eye.

Larger eye

Pull tight

ROUND TURN AND TWO HALF-HITCHES
Ties rope to a fixed point.
Start by winding the rope twice around a fixed point.

REEF KNOT, OR SQUARE KNOT
Flat knot used for tying reefing lines.

FIGURE OF EIGHT, OR STOP KNOT
Prevents rope from slipping through blocks.

LEFT-HAND BOWLINE
Keeps rope end out of the eye.

Rolling Hitch When a big override causes a sheet to be jammed on a winch, use a rolling hitch to attach a rope to the jammed sheet, between the sail and the winch. Take the tail of the rope to another winch and winch it in, thereby releasing the strain on the jammed sheet and allowing it to be easily cleared.

Sheet Bend The correct method of creating a sheet bend knot – which is used for tying ropes of different diameters together – as well as how to belay a rope around a cleat are also illustrated below.

It is wise to practise all the essential knots. Rope offcuts or damaged sheets are ideal for this.

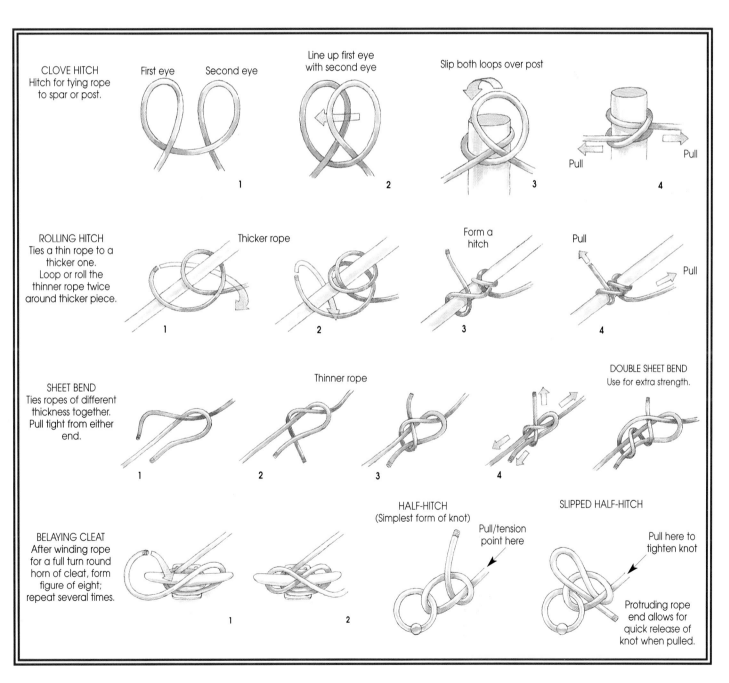

CLOVE HITCH
Hitch for tying rope to spar or post.

First eye   Second eye

Line up first eye with second eye

Slip both loops over post

Pull   Pull

1   2   3   4

ROLLING HITCH
Ties a thin rope to a thicker one. Loop or roll the thinner rope twice around thicker piece.

Thicker rope

Form a hitch

Pull   Pull

1   2   3   4

SHEET BEND
Ties ropes of different thickness together. Pull tight from either end.

Thinner rope

DOUBLE SHEET BEND
Use for extra strength.

1   2   3   4

BELAYING CLEAT
After winding rope for a full turn round horn of cleat, form figure of eight; repeat several times.

1   2

HALF-HITCH
(Simplest form of knot)

Pull/tension point here

SLIPPED HALF-HITCH

Pull here to tighten knot

Protruding rope end allows for quick release of knot when pulled.

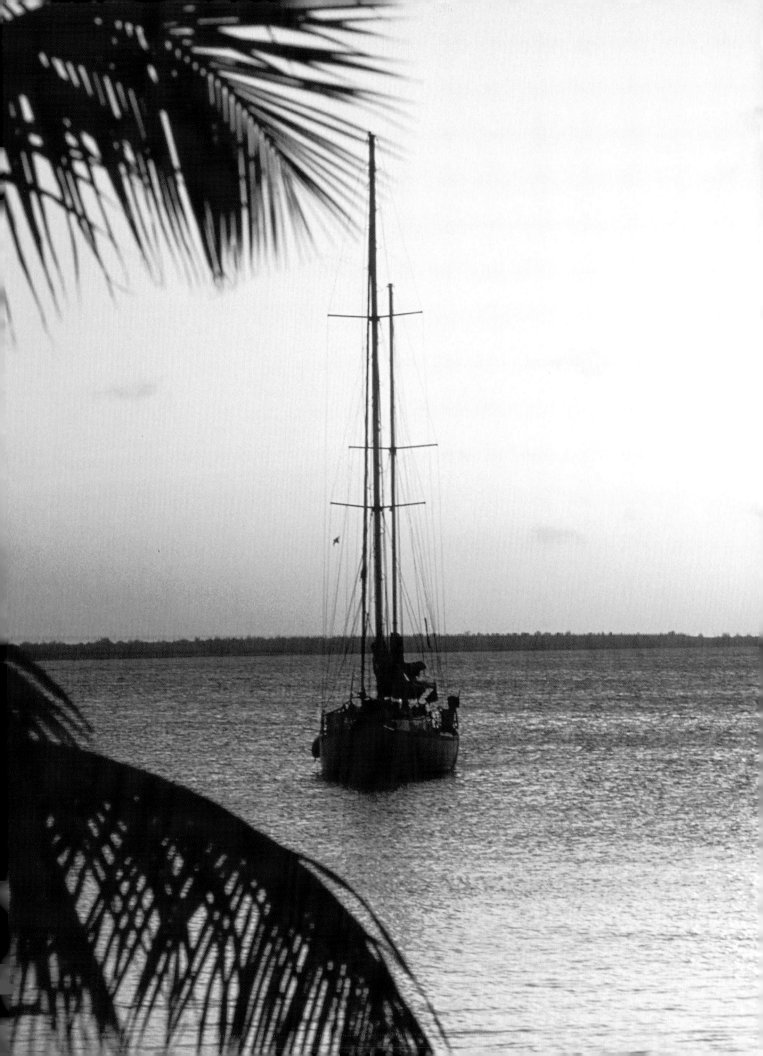

CRUISING
DESTINATIONS

Once you have acquired the necessary sailing skills, the ocean is your playground. You could choose to follow the trade winds around the world, or opt to spend time exploring a small section of coastline.

When planning your route, obtain cruising guides for the area to which you are bound. Most guides contain information such as the coordinates of harbours, the radio frequencies for contacting port authorities, the availability and cost of visitors' berths, what size boats can be accommodated, offshore anchorages and water depth, clearing customs, and whether water, fuel and other facilities (such as a chandlery, shops, laundromat, etc.) are available.

Staying at a full-service marina usually incurs costs on a daily basis. If you can't afford a long stay, plan to berth for a few days when you arrive in a new country to enable you to get a feel for the place and investigate alternative moorings.

During peak holiday season, particularly in the Caribbean and Mediterranean, you may have difficulty obtaining a berth or mooring at the most popular marinas. If you are determined to visit a particular place, book well in advance.

An easy way of cruising is to bareboat charter. Most of the big charter companies, such as Sunsail and the Moorings, have bases in the best cruising grounds. International yachting magazines will certainly list all the major charter companies active in the areas you are interested in.

Opposite *A tropical sunset, a deserted island, the sound of waves gently lapping against the hull, a warm breeze and a cool drink in your hand – this represents the picture-perfect image of cruising.*

BAREBOAT CHARTERING

Although you don't have the freedom to wander the high seas at will, there are many advantages to bareboat chartering, not least of which is the time factor. Cruising in your own boat means either staying close to home, or taking weeks, even months off work to cross the oceans to reach your destination.

With chartering, you fly in, make your way to the marina and within a few hours you can be under way. Some of the most obvious advantages are:

• You don't have capital tied up in your own boat.
• You can complete a cruise during your annual leave.
• Charter boats are generally in good condition and fully equipped. All the necessary charts will be on board and the charter company will help with advice on route planning.
• In the case of equipment or mechanical failure, the charter company is on hand to answer your VHF call and repair or replace the item concerned.
• You don't have to worry about maintenance and the associated costs.
• The boat is fully insured.

Below and opposite Chartering *offers the pleasures of cruising but none of the day-to-day problems of boat-owning.*

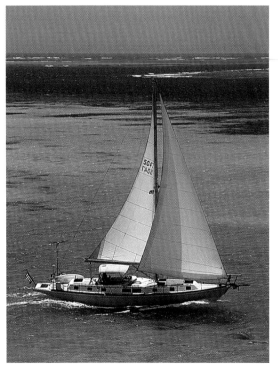

Selecting a charter company

Locating a good charter company is the key to having a wonderful holiday. There is nothing to beat word of mouth, so ask at your local yacht club for recommendations from happy customers.

Most reputable charter companies advertise in the yachting press, and there are specialist magazines aimed at the cruising and charter markets. The Internet is also a good resource for locating information on overseas-based companies.

Among the questions to ask are the following:

• If the charter company is European based, is it a member of the Association of Fully Bonded Sailing Companies? Membership offers guarantees and financial protection for clients.
• What type of fleet do they operate? Popular makes of charter craft include Gib'sea, Beneteau, Bavaria, and Jeanneau for monohulls; Robertson & Caine and Voyage Yachts for catamarans.

When chartering, there are a few simple rules worth observing, as they make life at sea more pleasant for you and for your fellow sailors.

• Obey local rules for anchoring, particularly where there is coral, as damage from anchors and chains may take decades to recover.
• Avoid problems with storing luggage on board by using soft carry-alls, not hard suitcases.
• Do not dump tins, plastics or anything not totally biodegradable into the sea. Store garbage in plastic bags and dispose of it in an appropriate area ashore. The same rule as for all wilderness areas applies: if in doubt, pack it out.
• In a marina or crowded anchorage, avoid late night parties that keep other people awake.

Charter boat ownership

Have you ever wondered how the charter companies are financed and how they raise the capital to buy fleets of brand new boats?

Well, many of the boats for hire are privately owned. Most of the charter companies have schemes whereby for a deposit of between 25 and 50 per cent, boat owners get income from their craft's charter activities plus a free annual charter holiday. After an agreed period, usually four to five years, ownership of the boat reverts to the owner.

Many people take this opportunity to obtain a boat at today's prices, for delivery in the future, while others do it for investment purposes, often selling the boat when the time period is up and reinvesting the money. If you've ever wished to own a cruising yacht, it is certainly worth investigating.

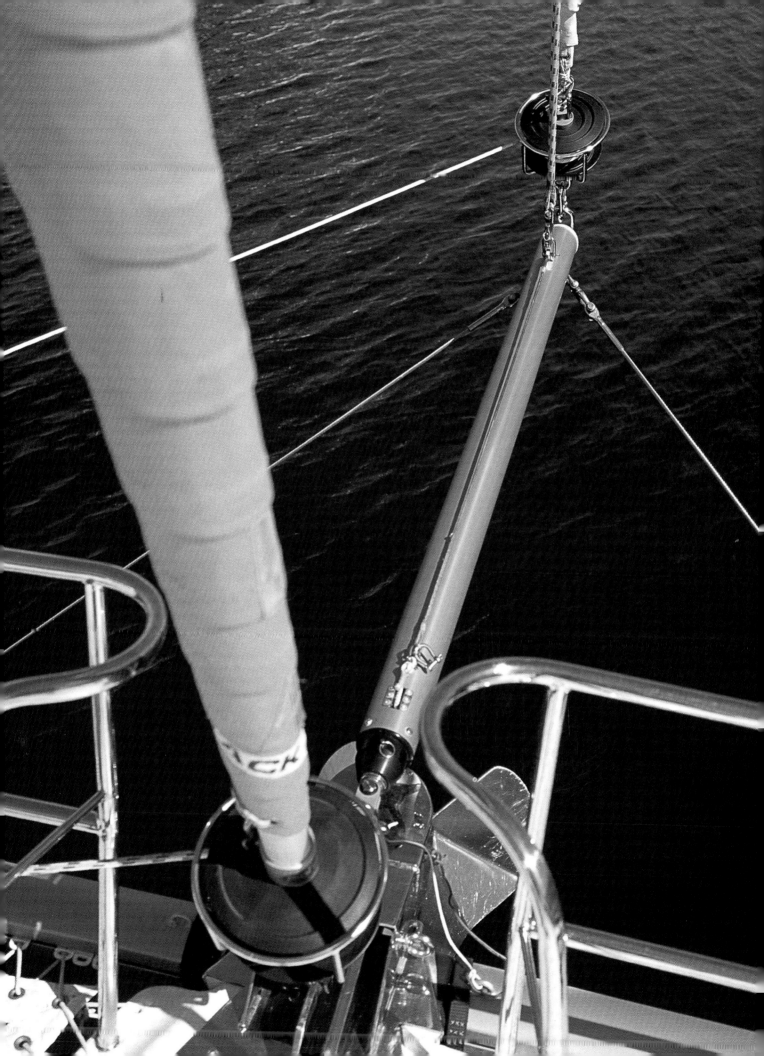

ROUTE PLANNING

Route planning across oceans is comparatively easy, as the vagaries of the prevailing winds are known on most routes. There are preferred times for leaving most places, while periods of poor weather are well documented, so you can easily avoid them.

Once you have arrived in your chosen area, you may find it hard to decide where to go, particularly in those cruising grounds that offer a wide choice of harbours and sheltered anchorages. Local weather and water conditions may determine your routes, as you discover lee shores or shallow waters, or learn when the wind is likely to switch direction, facilitating a passage from one island or harbour to another.

There are good cruising guides for every part of the world, and selecting the right ones will depend on where you sail and how long you plan to be at sea. Two reference books worth having are the British Admiralty publication *Ocean Passages*, and *World Cruising Routes* by yachtsman Jimmy Cornell.

Following the trade winds

Unless you are an experienced sailor, it is always best to follow one of the classic trade wind routes if you are crossing oceans. The trade winds blow year in and year out, varying in strength and direction from time to time, and you will generally have a trouble-free downwind ride.

The trade winds blow towards the equator from the northeast and southeast, creating ideal sailing conditions for boats travelling from Europe or Africa to the Caribbean, from the west coast of the USA or Central America across the Pacific, or from northern Australia across the Indian Ocean.

This 'low-latitude sailing' takes place in the tropics and subtropics, in the warm, balmy weather that is synonymous with vacation cruising.

The trade winds are the key to a traditional round-the-world cruise. If you start from the UK or Europe, drop down to the Canaries, then pick up the northeast trades which will take you across the Atlantic Ocean to the Caribbean or on to the Panama Canal.

Below Trade winds are prevailing winds that blow toward the equator from the northeast and southeast. They are caused by hot air rising at the equator and the consequent movement of air from north and south to take its place. The doldrums, an area of unpredictable calms, lie at their convergence. The winds are deflected to the west because of the earth's west to east rotation. The trade wind belts move about 5° to the north and south with the seasons.

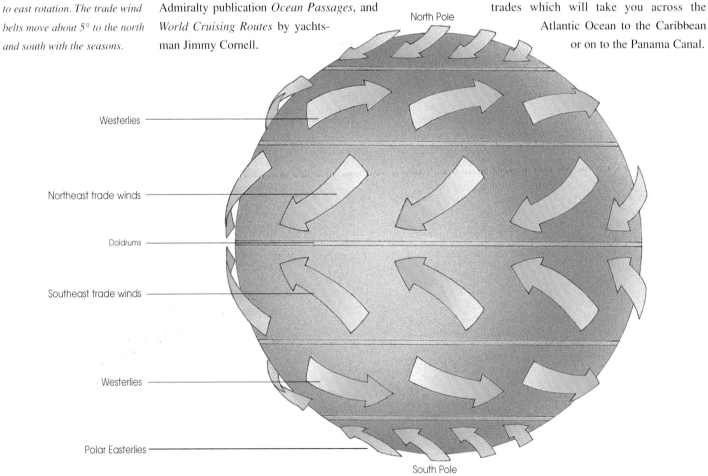

North Pole

Westerlies

Northeast trade winds

Doldrums

Southeast trade winds

Westerlies

Polar Easterlies

South Pole

From Cape Town, South Africa, pick up the south east trades to the mid-Atlantic islands of St Helena and Ascension, before heading for the Caribbean and the Panama Canal. Alternatively, after passing Ascension, you could turn northeast for Europe.

Once through the Panama Canal, you could cross the equator and pick up the southeast trades to the Galápagos, French Polynesia and the other South Pacific islands before going on to New Zealand. Heading north from Panama, the northeast trades will take you via Hawaii across the North Pacific.

From New Zealand, sail across the Tasman Sea to Australia then work your way up the east coast and the Great Barrier Reef before using the southeast trades to cross the Indian Ocean, perhaps via Mauritius and Réunion. From here, make for Durban or Richards Bay on the east coast of South Africa, or continue south to Cape Town.

Alternatively, sail northwest across the Indian Ocean via the Maldives or Seychelles and transit the Red Sea and Suez Canal into the Mediterranean. (This has become a problem route in recent years because of reported acts of piracy in the Red Sea.)

The basic rule with cruising is to look for routes that have the fewest headwinds combined with the greatest number of following winds. Naturally, during their seasons, you should avoid sailing in areas where hurricanes, cyclones or typhoons occur.

Choosing the correct sails

Sailing downwind (with the wind behind you) is about making the correct sail choice for your boat. Many people sail the trade wind routes under a fast rig comprising the mainsail and a poled-out jib. This requires concentration, due to the risk of an accidental gybe. It can also cause chafing where the mainsail touches the shrouds.

If you are prepared to travel more slowly, then you can dispense with the mainsail and set a second jib. Steering will be easy with both jibs poled out and either an automatic pilot (auto-helm) or self-steering gear can be used.

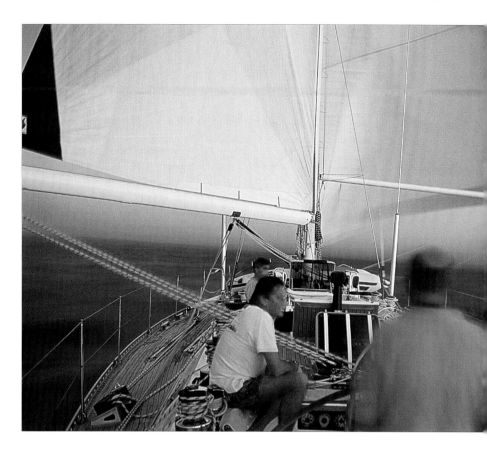

Cruising multihulls present a different problem with downwind sailing. The mainsail normally can't be eased out enough to run far off the wind because the stays are led very far aft. This gives good support for the mast, reduces compression and eliminates the need for backstays and runners, but it also means that the mainsail can only be used for beating and reaching. Many multihulls sail the trade wind routes with the mainsail permanently lowered, relying on just the jib or spinnaker.

The jib on its own is a bit slow for most conditions, so choose a combination of sails: a jib for heavy conditions and a spinnaker for lighter winds. Both can easily be controlled by autopilot or wind vane steering gear. (Before throwing up your hands in horror at the suggestion of a spinnaker, a cruising chute packed in a snuffer, and set without a pole being tacked down on the weather hull, is very easy to use and to douse in a hurry.)

Above *Good route planning is about making the best use of winds.* Le Maripier *has set a poled-out jib to catch every bit of breeze.*

Overleaf *When it comes to planning voyages across the oceans, proper nautical charts are essential, but a world atlas or basic map is nevertheless a good starting point.*

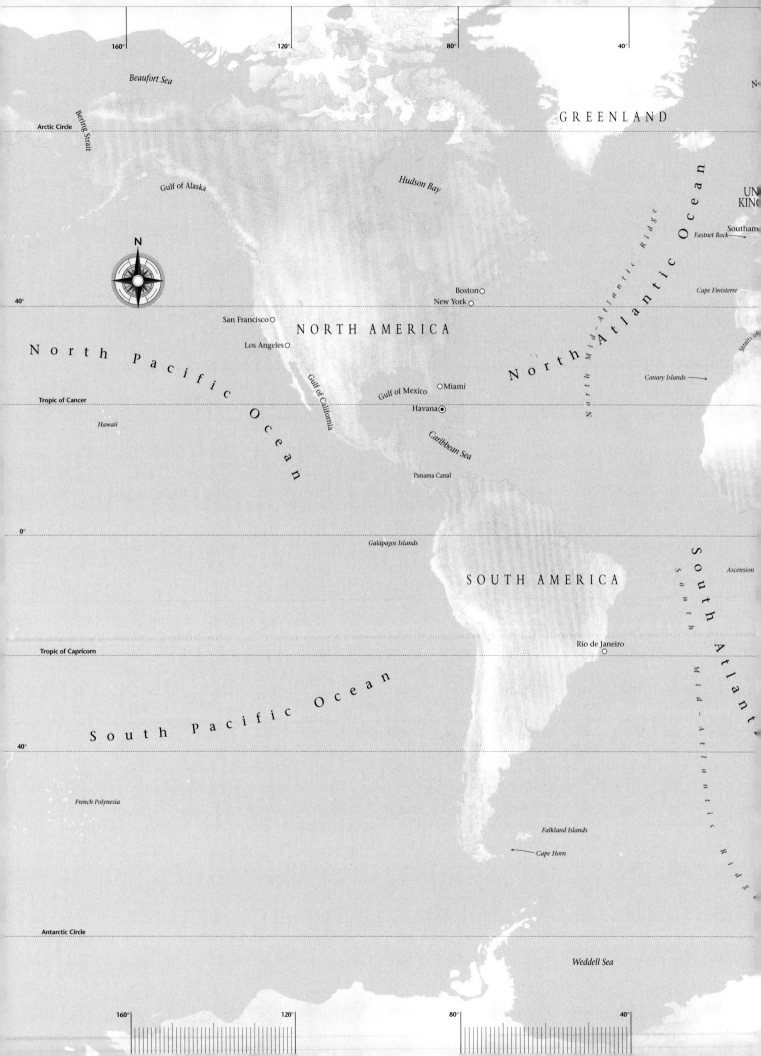

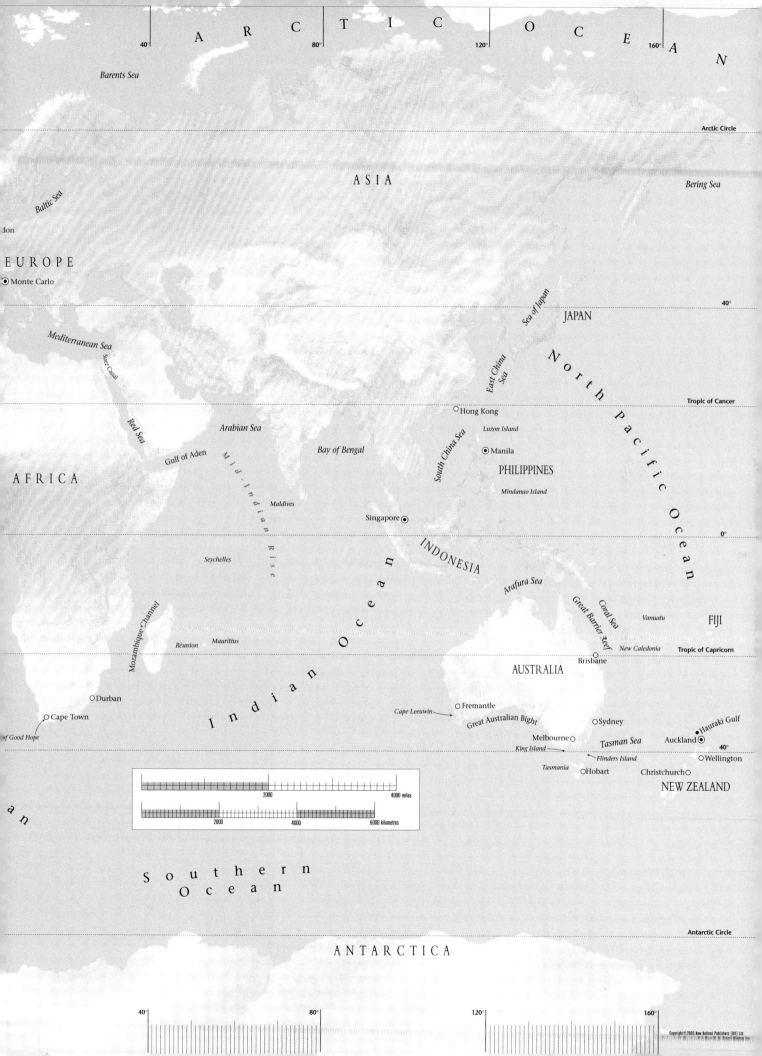

Barents Sea

ASIA

Bering Sea

Baltic Sea

Arctic Circle

EUROPE

⊙ Monte Carlo

40°

Mediterranean Sea

JAPAN

Sea of Japan

Suez Canal

East China Sea

Tropic of Cancer

Red Sea

Arabian Sea

Bay of Bengal

○ Hong Kong

Luzon Island

AFRICA

Gulf of Aden

South China Sea

⊙ Manila

North Pacific Ocean

Maldives

PHILIPPINES

Mindanao Island

Singapore ⊙

0°

Seychelles

INDONESIA

Arafura Sea

Coral Sea

Vanuatu

FIJI

Great Barrier Reef

Indian Ocean

Mozambique Channel

Réunion   *Mauritius*

New Caledonia

Tropic of Capricorn

Brisbane ○

AUSTRALIA

○ Durban

○ Fremantle

Cape Leeuwin

Great Australian Bight

○ Sydney

● Hauraki Gulf

○ Cape Town

Melbourne ○

Tasman Sea

Auckland ⊙

40°

of Good Hope

King Island

Flinders Island

○ Wellington

Tasmania

○ Hobart

Christchurch ○

NEW ZEALAND

			2000		4000 miles

	2000		4000		6000 kilometres

S o u t h e r n
O c e a n

Antarctic Circle

A N T A R C T I C A

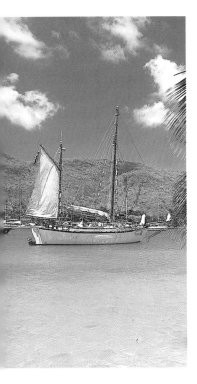

Above *A traditional ketch at anchor in Admiralty Bay off Bequia, the largest island in the Grenadines.*

Opposite *Marigot Bay on St Lucia, in the Windward Islands, is typical of the sheltered bays that attract yachts to the Lesser Antilles.*

THE CARIBBEAN

The Caribbean stretches from Trinidad and Tobago in the southeast through the chain of islands that make up the Lesser Antilles, then curves north towards Antigua, Barbuda and the Virgin Islands before turning west towards Puerto Rico, Dominican Republic, Jamaica and Cuba. To the west, lie Mexico's Yucatán Peninsula and Central America, while Colombia and Venezuela form the southern boundary.

Situated in the Atlantic, rather than the Caribbean itself, the islands and cays of the Bahamas are within easy reach of cruising yachts setting out from Miami, Fort Lauderdale or the Florida Keys.

Extending from latitude 10° north to about 25° north, the entire area has a delightful tropical climate. The region is swept by the northeast trade winds virtually all year round and would be ideal for nonstop sailing if it were not for hurricanes, which can occur anywhere in the Caribbean from June to November (mid-summer through fall).

Hurricane activity is well forecast and all tropical storm systems are monitored from their initial formation until they disintegrate over the Atlantic. Sailing during hurricane season should be carefully planned, and many private boats and charter fleets choose to lay up during this period.

Caribbean cruising is legendary among yachtsmen. If you have the time and money, you can island hop, cruising from marina to marina or stopping off at one of the many good anchorages scattered throughout the region. You can spend every night in a different place for several months and will only have scratched the surface. A bonus for novice sailors is that tides are slight, navigation is easy and you can usually see the destination for which you are bound.

Chartering is well-established here, and Sunsail, the Moorings and Voyage Yachts are among the many companies who have made it into a thriving industry. Most of the big charter operations have bases on more than one island. They all offer a variety of boat sizes to suit your sailing skills and the size of your group, as well as a choice between monohull and catamaran, both of which have their good and bad points.

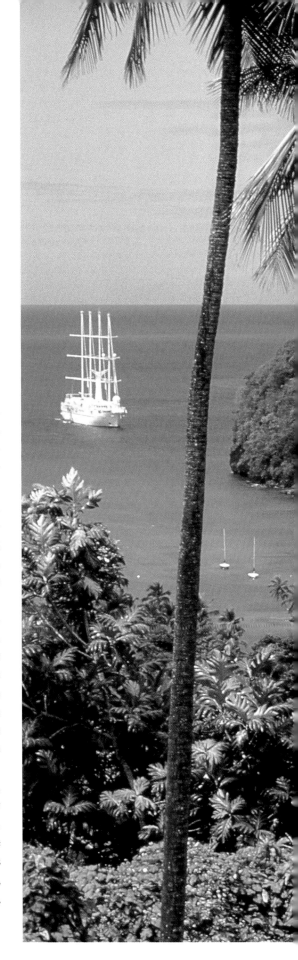

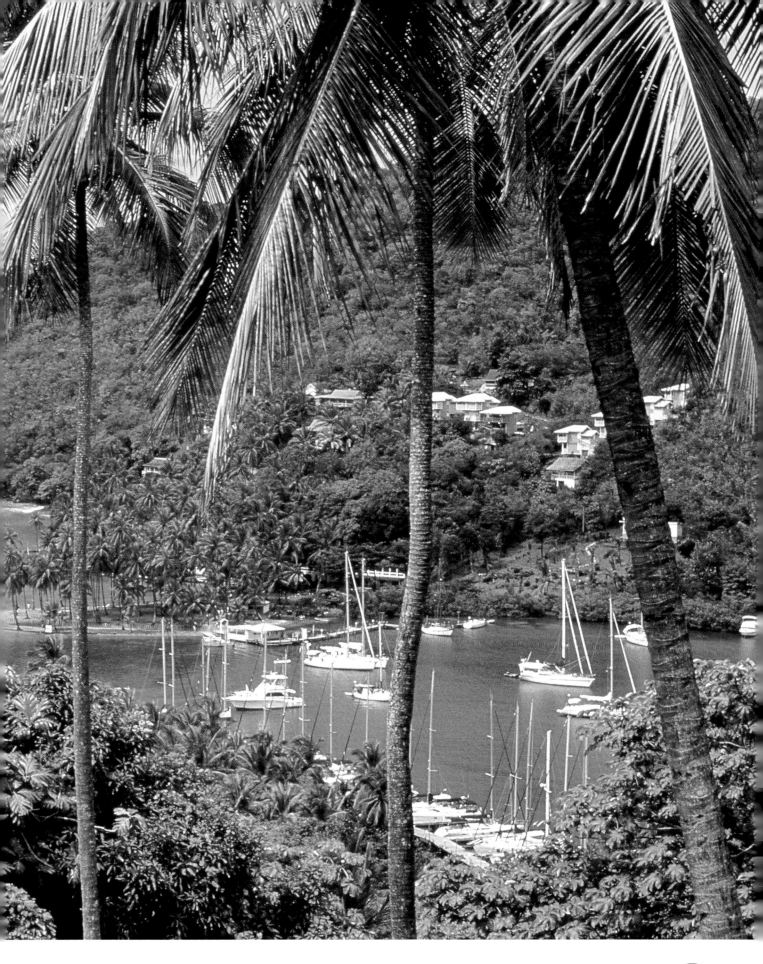

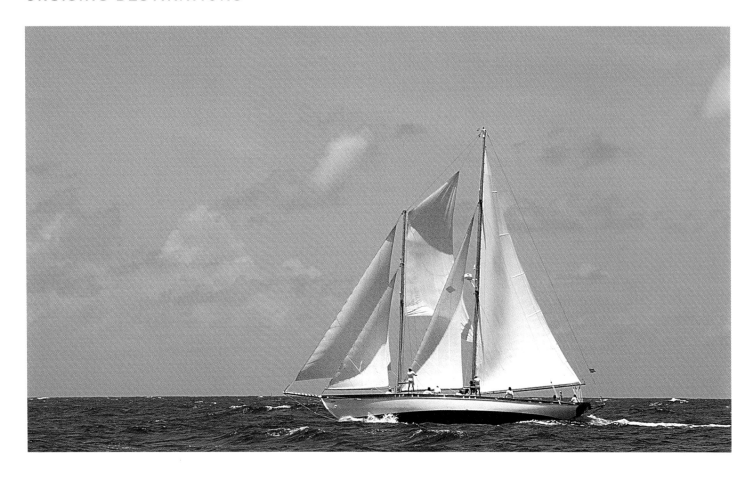

Above *A traditional schooner revels in the trade wind conditions off Antigua.*

Opposite *Enjoying a sunset cruise off St John in the US Virgin Islands.*

Monohulls sail to windward well, but the deep draught limits your mooring options. In an anchorage exposed to the trade winds or an ocean swell, monohulls tend to roll whereas catamarans do not. The catamaran's draught means it can be run into most shallow areas, making it ideal for swimming, snorkelling and easy access ashore.

Once you have made your choice of boat, there are many sailing options. Most islands are in sight of one another and navigation is easy. The winds are fairly constant and the northeast trade winds generally blow at moderate strength day after day.

Most Caribbean nations depend on tourism, and festivals and other events take place throughout the year. For sailors, race weeks are held at yacht clubs on many of the islands and visitors are welcome.

The Caribbean is a scuba diver's paradise, but there is also plenty of good snorkelling for those who are not certified divers.

Antigua and Barbuda

The Leeward Islands, in the Lesser Antilles, comprise Antigua, Barbuda, St Kitts, Nevis, St Maarten, Saba, St Eustatius, St Barthélémy, Anguilla and Monserrat. Situated where the Atlantic meets the Caribbean Sea, the surrounding waters are often turbulent.

Antigua is separated from Barbuda by about 48km (30 miles) of rough water. Both islands offer many safe and sheltered anchorages, giving them a deserved reputation as a cruising paradise. Land-based tourism centres around their 365 beaches.

English Harbour, a picturesque natural anchorage, is the home of the Antigua Sailing Week regatta, one of the most popular events on the international sailing calendar (see p133). Combining long-distance and round-the-buoys races with parties, food festivals and other activities, it attracts yachties from all over the world. If you plan to cruise in this area, do so in late April so that you can be part of this event.

Virgin Islands

About 100 islands make up this northernmost group of the Leeward Islands in the Antilles, about 95km (60 miles) west of Puerto Rico.

Discovered by Christopher Columbus in 1493 and named for St Ursula and her 11,000 virgin followers, they comprise two quite distinct territories, the US Virgin Islands (USVI) – St Thomas, St Croix and St John – and the British Virgin Islands (BVI) – Tortola, Virgin Gorda, Anegada and Jost van Dykes.

The islands, which were once the haunt of pirates such as Henry Morgan and the infamous Blackbeard, are the remains of a subterranean volcanic mountain plateau, giving rise to deep waters close inshore and thousands of sheltered bays and coves.

The climate is good, with hot, humid summers. Hurricanes can occur from September to January.

The Virgin Islands offer some of the best sailing in the Caribbean. Red Hook, on St Thomas in the USVI, is a key base for charter boats, while Tortola fulfills the same role in the BVI. Anegada, which lies 40km (25 miles) northeast of Tortola, has the largest barrier reef in the eastern Caribbean (the third largest in the world) making it a popular dive destination.

Tourism is well developed, with resorts catering for all tastes and pockets. St Croix and St Thomas are easily reached by international flights from most major US airports. Flights from the UK to the BVI are usually routed via San Juan in Puerto Rico.

Barbados

Barbados, the easternmost island in the Caribbean, is one of the Windward Islands. Although tiny, its 97km (60 miles) of coral coastline has plenty to offer the passing sailor. The rugged cliffs of the east coast are pounded by the Atlantic Ocean, but the rest of the island has endless white beaches and calm waters. The cooling northeast trade winds keep temperatures between 23 and 29°C (75–85°F). Tropical rainstorms occur from June to October.

Despite the high population density, the people are fun-loving and friendly, but understanding the unique island dialect takes some getting used to.

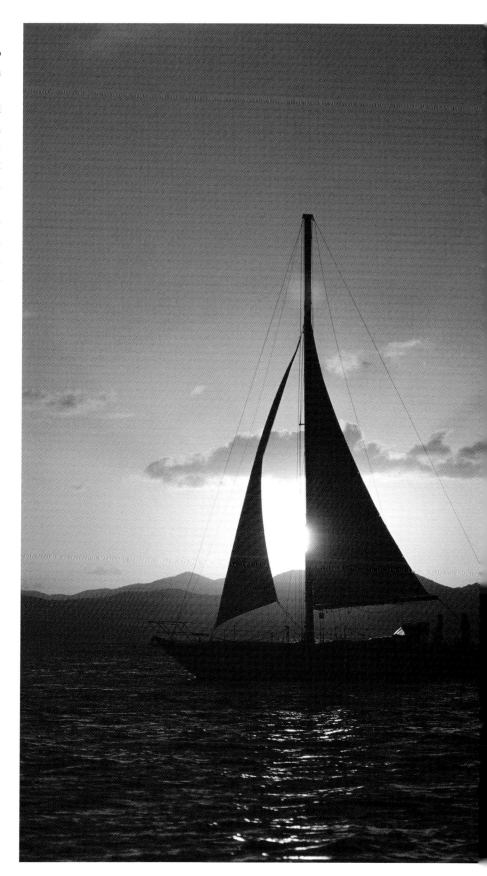

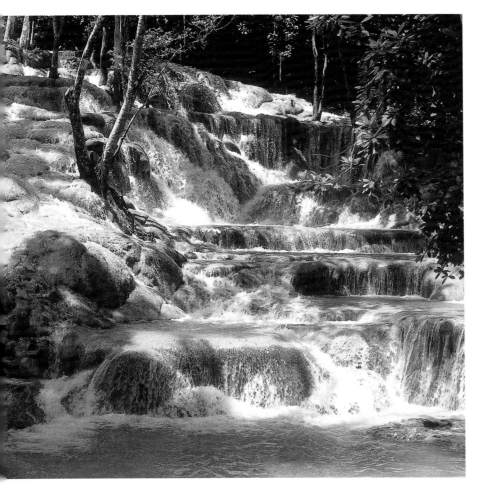

Henry Morgan (who changed his ways and went on to become a governor of Jamaica).

Just offshore of the popular tourist town of Port Antonio, on the northeast coast, is Navy Island, which has a yacht club and some beautiful beaches. At the opposite end of the island is Montego Bay, a tourist hub that is famous for its white sand beaches and the annual Reggae Sunsplash, a week-long music festival held each August.

Bahamas

Just 80km (50 miles) from Florida, these 'islands in the stream' were made famous by Ernest Hemingway, who lived on Bimini. The Gulf Stream begins its journey here, making the 23 inhabited islands and thousands of unpopulated cays and islets a paradise for sailors and game fisherman alike.

Despite the Bahamas' popularity with tourists, it is possible to find secluded anchorages. Many of the islands' white sand beaches are deserted because they are only accessible from the water.

Above *Waterfalls such as the Dunn's River Falls are common near Ocho Rios on Jamaica's northern shore.*

Right *Charter catamarans share moorings with luxury motor cruisers in the Bahamas.*

Opposite *At anchor off Mexico's tranquil Caribbean coast.*

Jamaica and the Cayman Islands

Sea breezes mingle with the scent of flowers, coconut oil, Blue Mountain coffee and rum punch to herald your arrival on Jamaica, the third largest island in the Caribbean, 130km (80 miles) south of Cuba.

Between Jamaica and Cuba lie the Caymans, three tiny islands (the largest only 44km/28 miles long), with a reputation as one of the world's top dive sites.

Warm seas, sandy beaches, exotic cocktails and the reggae beat embody the laid-back island style that attracts yachties and land-based travellers alike. At 18° north, the climate is typically hot and humid all year round (averaging 28°C/82°F at the coast), relieved by steady breezes from the north. Tropical storms occur during hurricane season, from July to October.

Visiting sailors are welcome at the Royal Jamaica Yacht Club in Port Royal, once a haven for pirates and buccaneers like Edward 'Blackbeard' Teach and

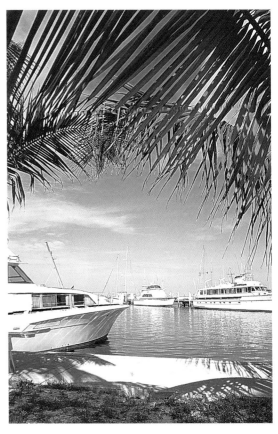

All the main Bahamian islands hold regattas, usually in the late summer, as well as noncompetitive sailing events, which are inevitably accompanied by parties and barbeques. Chartering is a big business in the Bahamas, with most companies operating out of Nassau, the capital.

Among the islands favoured by yachtsmen are the Berry Islands, a group of 30 secluded cays covering 30 km² (12 sq miles). Call at Port Nelson on Rum Cay, a town which is reputed to have derived its name from the wreck of a West Indian rum-runner, and spend time on the pink sands of Harbour Island, just offshore of Eleuthera.

Don't forget to look for the elusive green flash – a natural tropical phenomenon that occurs on cloudless days just after the sun sinks into the sea. If you are fortunate, you'll see a band of brilliant green light flash across the horizon. It's rare, but it happens.

Mexico

Jutting into the Caribbean, the Yucatán peninsula and the coral-ringed islands of Cozumel and Isla Mujeres are popular tourist destinations. These ancient Mayan strongholds are rich with Mexican heritage and it is worth spending time ashore to visit some of the ruins of this once dominant culture.

Isla Mujeres (Island of Women) is 11km (7 miles) from the resort city of Cancún. Anchor off the sheltered western and southern shores and explore the small island on foot or by hired moped.

If scuba diving is your thing, Cozumel is a must. Palancar Reef, the world's second longest, extends for 37km (23 miles) offshore. It is rich in tropical fish, underwater caves and tunnels. Experienced divers head for the Maracaibo, Paraíso and Yocab reefs for drift diving in light currents.

Daytime temperatures in the Yucatán average 26°C (79°F) on the coast, hotter in the interior. Rain falls from April to May and September to January. Hurricanes can occur between July and October.

Many cruising sailors bypass Mexico in favour of the better-known Caribbean islands, but if you've 'been there, done that', perhaps it is time to explore some alternative anchorages.

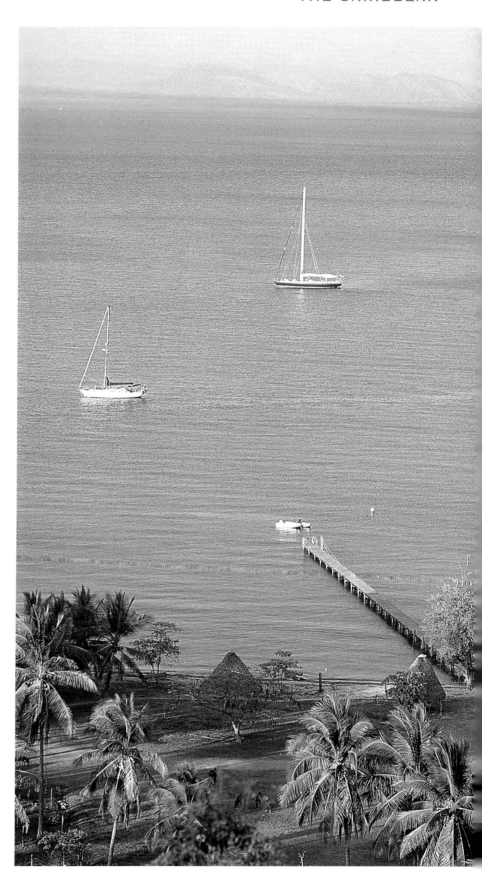

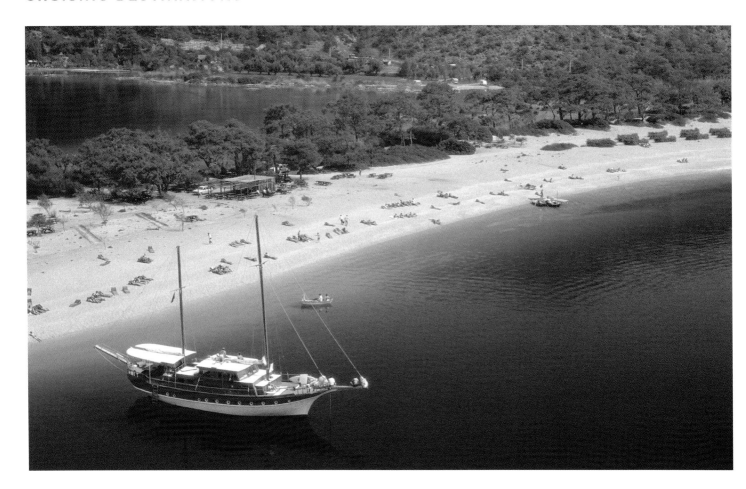

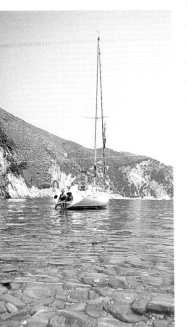

MEDITERRANEAN SEA

Throughout the summer, the entire Mediterranean coast is an excellent cruising ground, from Spain and the Balearic isles in the west, via France and Italy, to Greece and Turkey in the east. Adventurous sailors can also explore Morocco, Algeria, Libya and Egypt on the African coast. Many yachties say they never want to sail anywhere else.

Navigation is easy and the tide is virtually non-existent. Passages between anchorages are short, most of the sailing can be accomplished in daylight and you can be snugly tied up or anchored by nightfall. People tend to go ashore for their evening meal, thus avoiding the need to prepare cooked meals on board. Best of all, 'the Med' is an area to which you can safely take even a nonenthusiastic sailor.

Charter companies are well established in the Med, particularly in Greece and Turkey. Charter a bareboat for a week or two and experience the joy of cruising without the responsibility of owning a boat.

If you are new to chartering, you could consider a flotilla cruise. The flotilla leader plans the route and will ensure you understand where the next rendezvous is. You sail independently during the day and meet up with the flotilla group at a predetermined anchorage each evening.

In the Mediterranean, mooring is often stern-on to a wharf or jetty. You drop the bow anchor and then reverse in to the wharf, often a tight squeeze between two boats. The person handling the anchor-line must ease it out at just the right speed, and the helmsman must be reasonably competent at handling a boat going astern under power.

When visiting popular ports in high season, try to arrive early so you can have your pick of the berths. Late arrivals may find that their chosen marina is full, leaving them to make alternative plans.

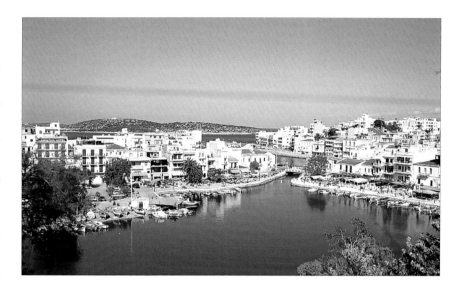

Greece

Greece and Turkey are the countries which come to people's minds when they think of chartering. The summer weather is delightful, with light sailing conditions and it is easy to find somewhere different to stop every night.

The more than 1400 Greek islands make up some 25,000 km² (10,000 sq miles), spread over two seas. Although they are grouped together for administrative and tourism purposes, each island has an individual identity that is as much cultural as it is physical.

High mid-summer temperatures are made bearable by the *meltémi*, a northerly wind that begins at dawn as a breeze and escalates during the day, before dying down in the evening. Sailors are particularly affected and, if you spend the night in a north-facing bay, you need to set sail early or risk being trapped until the wind abates.

In the relatively shallow Aegean Sea, strong prevailing winds can create hazardous sea conditions which make sailing near rocky shores difficult.

CORFU

Cypress trees and olive groves give the seven Ionian islands, Zante (Zákinthos), Cephalonia (Kefaloniá), Ithaca (Itháki), Lefkás (Lefkáda), Páxos (Paxí), Corfu (Kérkyra) and the southerly Kythira, an Italian feel. Here the summers are hot and humid, with hazy skies and gentle breezes, while winters can be cold and wet,

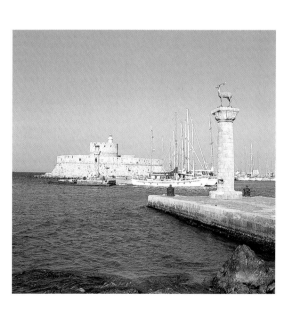

with strong winds from the south and northeast. Tides are almost nonexistent and navigation is easy.

Corfu boasts some of the best beaches in Greece and, although popular with tourists, remains relatively unspoilt. Kondókali, north of Corfu town, has a protected marina and an offshore island in Gouvia Bay.

For quieter anchorages, head for Barbáti, at the foot of Mt Pantokrator; Kalámi, once the home of writers Lawrence and Gerald Durrell; or Kouloúra, where life centres around the attractive old harbour.

RHODES

Situated closer to Turkey than to mainland Greece, Rhodes is the largest of the Dodecanese chain. It is very popular with visitors, but it is possible to escape the crowds, particularly out of season.

Light *meltémi* breezes from the northwest provide mostly ideal sailing conditions. Navigation is by line of sight, but the shoreline is rocky, so take care when anchoring.

Explore Kámiros Skála, a fishing port with a small harbour, or sail to one of the islands off Rhodes' west coast, Makrí, Strongíli or Chálki, once the centre of a thriving natural sponge industry. Beyond Kritinía, the slopes of Mt Atáviros fall steeply into the sea.

The ruins of Kastrou Monólithos, a Crusader castle, stand out atop the rock pinnacle of Monópetros. Further along the coast, Apolákia Bay has numerous deserted sand and shingle beaches.

Above *Houses line the quayside at Agios Nikolaos on Zante, one of the Ionian islands.*

Below left *Bronze deer mark the entrance to the harbour at Mandraki, on Rhodes.*

Opposite top *In Turkey, many wooden gulets, like this one off Olü Deniz, operate on a crewed charter basis.*

Opposite bottom *A sugar-scoop stern makes it easy to get out of the water after a swim.*

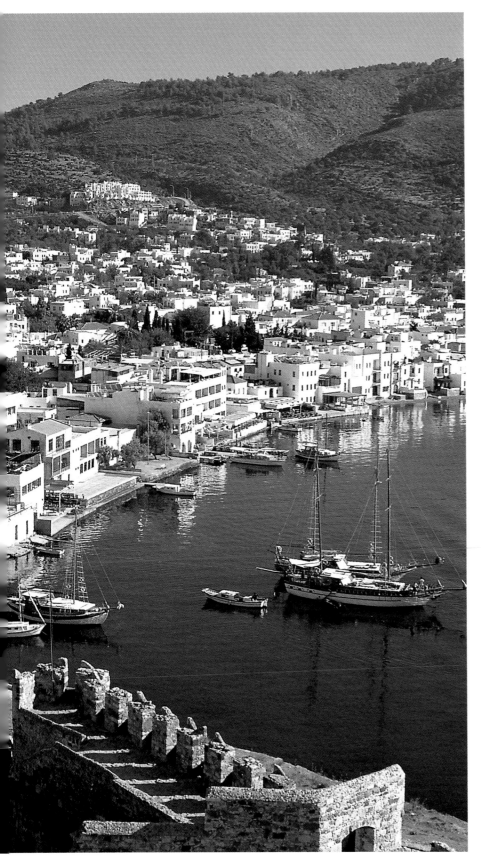

Turkey

Turkey, an historic meeting point between East and West, is a cultural and religious amalgam that has been forged across the centuries. In its modern incarnation, it still merges the ancient with the contemporary.

With extensive coastlines facing both the Aegean and Mediterranean seas, Turkey is a popular cruising destination and there are many bareboat charter companies operating in these waters.

The Aegean coast boasts numerous small islets and sheltered coves with warm aquamarine sea and sandy beaches, overlooked by olive groves, which attract the crowds to the most popular towns, such as Bodrum and Kusadasi.

The Castle of St Peter, which lies at the entrance to Bodrum harbour, was built by the Crusaders in the 15th century. It contains the Museum of Underwater Archaeology, a collection of treasures from the many vessels lost at sea along these coasts.

The ruins of three ancient cities, Ephesus, Troy and Pergamum, are found along the Aegean coast. If you have an interest in history or archaeology, it is worth making an effort to arrange excursions to one or more of these sites.

Many of the more remote beaches and coves in the western stretch of this coast can only be reached by boat. Resorts and sailing centres here include Marmaris, Fethiye and Koycegiz. Marmaris, which is reputed to have the finest natural harbour in the eastern Mediterranean, also has the largest marina in Turkey. It is a bustling town with good nightlife, making it a good base for charter cruisers.

North of Fethiye, in an area called the Turquoise Coast, the small port of Göçek, another charter base, nestles in a secluded bay. In the opposite direction is Ölüdeniz, a well-frequented anchorage with a spectacular lagoon and good swimming beaches.

Kas (Kos) has a pretty harbour and is known for its nightlife. Just off Kas is Kekova Island, where the remains of a Roman city are visible beneath the water.

En route to Antalya, visit the retreat of Olympos, where an eternal flame burns continually, thanks to natural gas escaping from the hillside. Antalya itself overlooks a wide bay and harbour.

Côte d' Azur

The coastline of Provence and the Cote d' Azur varies from rocky bays and inlets to sandy beaches, both natural and man-made. Summers are long and hot and winters cool and often rainy. The mistral, that famous cold, dry wind, funnels down the Rhône valley in winter, causing temperatures to drop and tempers to flare as it blasts the region for days on end.

Provence is a land bathed in sunshine and scented with herbs and lavender, where groves of olive trees vie for space with vineyards, and the Camargue's famous white horses and black bulls are as much a symbol as the bronzed bodies on the golden beaches of Cannes and Nice.

It is an expensive region and thrifty cruisers may prefer to bypass the trendy towns in favour of local fishing harbours, where prices are more realistic.

In Marseille, France's third-largest city and a major harbour, the old port is a sought-after mooring spot for visiting yachtsmen. Between Marseille and the village of Cassis, to the east, are the Calanques, a series of steep-sided bays and inlets tucked into the white limestone cliffs and often ending in beaches.

Martigues, a nearby harbour town with a small marina, has a medieval town centre with a variety of typical market stalls.

Explore one of the small islands off the French Riviera. Ile de Port-Cros and Ile de Porquerolles, off Hyères, are nature reserves, while on St Honorat, near Cannes, a fourth-century monastery is still home to a community of monks.

Nestling between the mountains and the Baie des Anges, Nice was first settled by the Romans in 154BC. The port is protected by a jetty which shelters yachts and luxury motor cruisers alike. From here, it is 108 nautical miles to Corsica, which offers an almost endless choice of excellent cruising.

To the northwest of the famous beaches of St Tropez is the medieval town of Grimaud and modern Port Grimaud, a marina village where canals have replaced roads and yachts are moored at the 'bottom of the garden'. The permanent resident population is boosted by a regular influx of summer yachties.

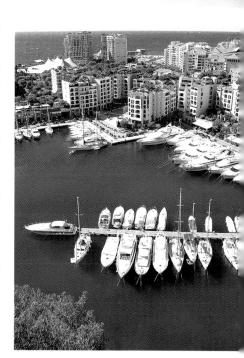

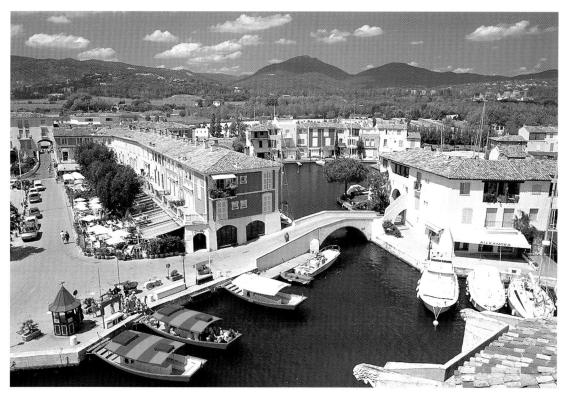

Above *Luxurious yachts and motor cruisers compete for space in Monaco, on the Côte d'Azur.*

Left *In the residential marina of Port Grimaud, canals link the homes, and boats are as much a feature as motor cars.*

Opposite *The ruins of the Castle of St Peter overlook the town of Bodrum, on Turkey's Aegean coast.*

Right *Puerto Banus, on the Costa del Sol, is an affluent and sophisticated resort town.*

Opposite *At Eivissa, Ibiza, the old town clings to the hill.*

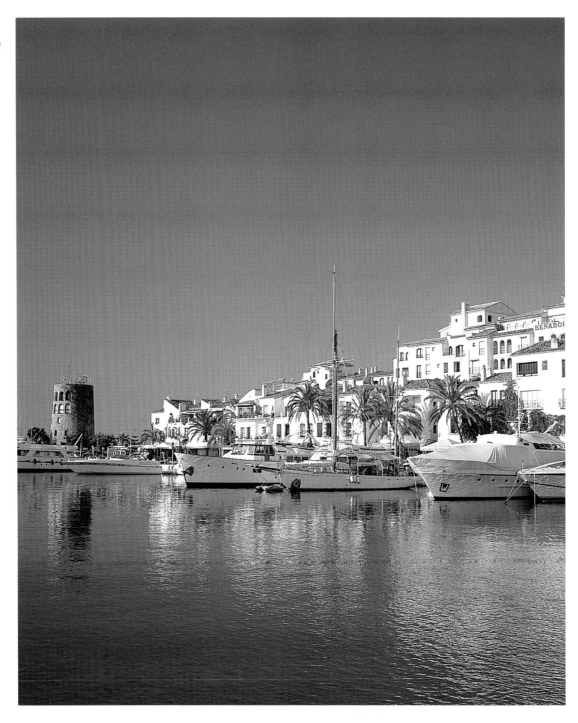

Costa del Sol and Gibraltar

Spain's 'sunshine coast', from Gibraltar in the west to Almería in the east, is one of Europe's top holiday destinations. This is a land of festivals and fiestas, where many towns celebrate their saint's day with a *romería*, or pilgrimage, to a holy spot.

The Costa del Sol embodies the essence of Spain, from its fragrant orange orchards and dappled olive groves to the heated rhythm of flamenco and the crisp dryness of a *fino* wine from Jerez.

Protected by mountain ranges, the summers on the coast are long and hot, with plenty of sunshine, low humidity and balmy evenings, while winters are mild. Rain can fall from December to March.

Just west of Marbella is Puerto Banus, a *pueblo*, or village-style port for the rich (if not famous), where the luxury vessels lining the marina are the stuff of dreams. Near Malaga is Torremolinos, a lively resort with two good beaches and a vibrant nightlife centred around Calle San Miguel.

Like Puerto Banus, many of the marinas along the Costa del Sol have shops, taverns and restaurants as well as accommodation. Enquire about moorings at Puerto Cabopino, located just outside Marbella, or at Benelmádena Puerto, Marina del Este in Granada province or La Duquesa towards Gibraltar.

Strategically positioned at the entrance to the Mediterranean, it is no wonder the citadel-like rock of Gibraltar has seen centuries of strife.

Today it is a British colony and an important naval base. Fast currents and deep water surround the rock, causing violent winds and storms, so take care when passing through the narrow channel of the Straits.

From Gibraltar, it is a short sail to Tangier in Morocco, or Ceuta, a Spanish enclave in North Africa.

Balearic Islands

The Balearic Isles (Mallorca, Menorca, Ibiza and Formentera) offer sunny summers, sparkling seas and white beaches cooled by sea breezes. The islands are a holiday playground, attracting thousands of tourists each year, many of whom come for the nightlife and world-famous clubs.

Mallorca's coastline is dramatic, with two huge bays, hundreds of hidden coves, and cliffs that plunge into the sea. Menorca has more accessible beaches and *calas*, or coves, while many of Ibiza's 56 small beaches are only accessible from the sea.

Seek the breeze along Mallorca's east coast as you explore tiny unspoilt bays, or seek a berth at a luxury marina on the Costa del Pins. On Menorca, drop anchor in the beautiful cove of Cala Santa Galdana, or moor at the quayside in the port of Cuitadella. Ibiza's tranquil southern shores are unspoilt; from here it is a short sail to Formentera, where it is easy to find a secluded cove to anchor for lunch, or for the night.

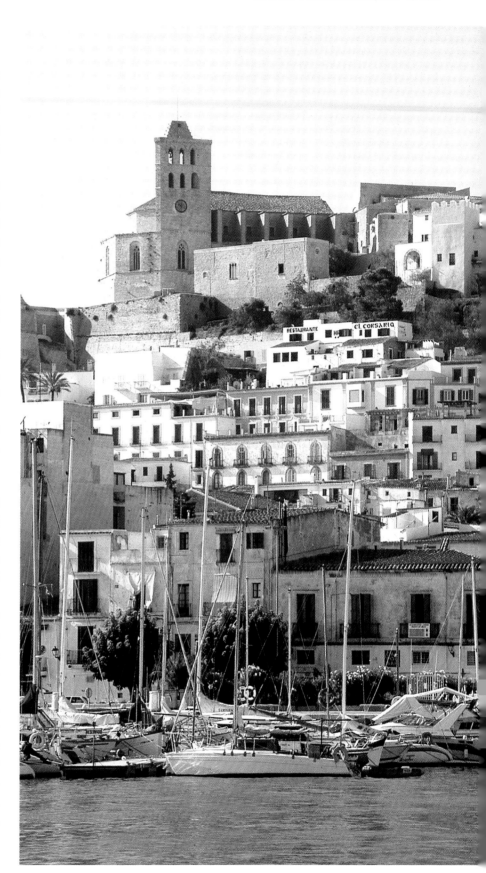

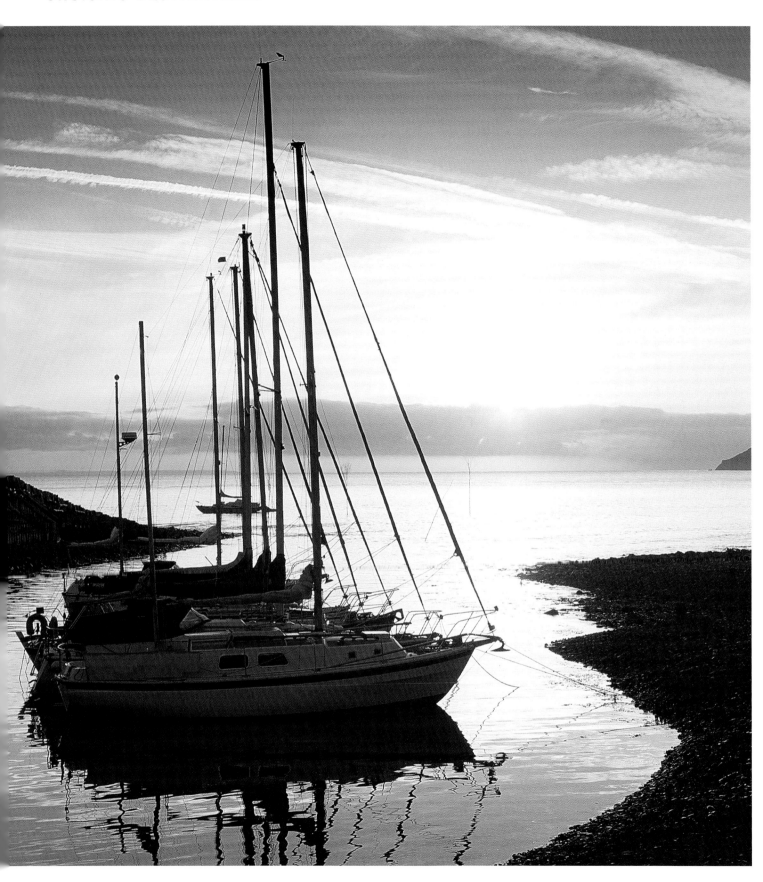

UNITED KINGDOM

Isle of Wight and the English Channel

The Isle of Wight and Cowes are synonymous with sailing worldwide. The Royal Yacht Squadron, one of the originators of yacht racing, is based here, and the turbulent waters of the Solent have been the proving ground for many top ocean-going sailors.

Although much of the focus is on the Cowes Week regatta and Round the Island Race held each August, as well as the biennial Admiral's Cup races, there are sailing activities on the island throughout the year.

There are a number of yacht clubs and marinas on the Isle of Wight, but most visiting cruisers head for Cowes itself, where the Royal Yacht Squadron, Island Sailing Club and Cowes Yacht Haven offer moorings within walking distance of the town centre. Berths can be scarce at peak times.

From the Isle of Wight it is a short sail to the Channel Islands, Jersey, Guernsey, Alderney and Sark, which lie within the sheltered waters of the Gulf of St Malo. St Helier is the only deep-water harbour on Jersey, but smaller boats can moor at drying harbours at St Aubin and Gorey. (The tidal range around Jersey can be as much as 12m/40ft at spring tide, but even the normal daily ebb and flow means that mooring or berthing requires extra care, so obtain local advice if you are unfamiliar with the area.)

Ireland

The seas surrounding the Emerald Isle offer a variety of interesting cruising options, particularly for those who prefer to combine sailing with time ashore.

Start at Dun Laoghaire (pronounced Dun Leary) in Dublin Bay, home of the Royal Irish Yacht Club, and make your way south to the natural harbour at Wexford. The southeast coast has some excellent beaches, particularly at Waterford and Tramore, where there is also a marina.

Situated on an estuary opening into the Atlantic, Cork, Ireland's third city, has a long maritime history. The Royal Cork Yacht Club is one of the oldest in the world. Like many other coastal towns in the southwest, Kinsale has a perfect natural harbour.

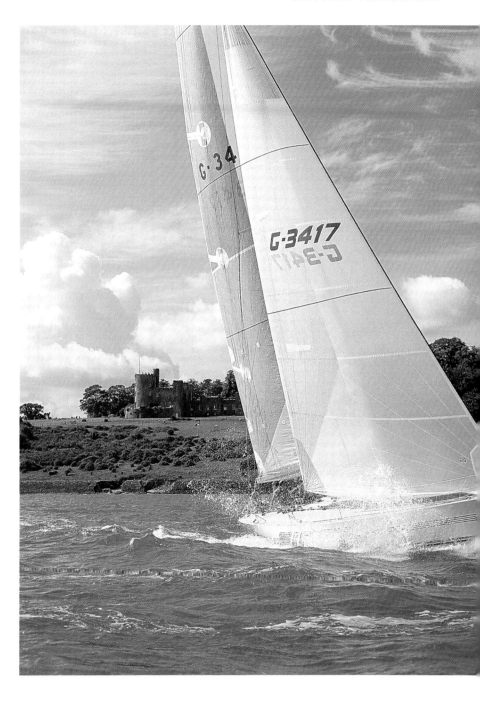

The southwest coast of Ireland is dotted with small islands and deeply indented bays. The Blasket Islands, just off the windswept Dingle peninsula, are the westernmost point in Europe. To the north, in county Clare, the imposing Cliffs of Moher stretch for 8km (5 miles) along the coast, rising 215m (705ft) above the sea. Across South Sound, the barren Aran Islands lie in the quiet waters of Galway Bay.

Above *The waters of the Solent, off the Isle of Wight, offer some challenging sailing.*

Opposite *At anchor on the tidal flats in one of the UK's many estuaries.*

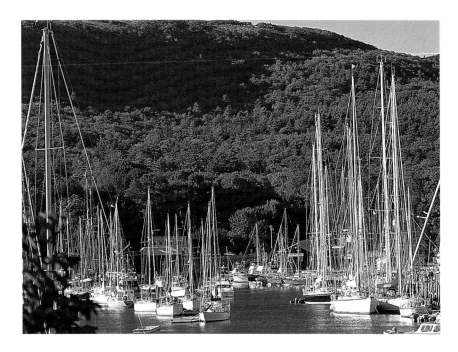

Above *The Maine coast, with its many inlets and secluded anchorages, makes a good summer cruising ground.*

Right *San Diego, in California, is a key centre for yachting on the US West Coast.*

Opposite *Brushed by the Gulf Stream, the warm, calm seas and coral reefs of the Bahamas provide exceptional cruising.*

THE USA

The USA offers a wide variety of cruising waters, from subtropical Florida in the south to cold Maine in the north. Both the East and West coasts, as well as the Great Lakes, are established cruising areas.

Intra-Coastal Waterway and Chesapeake Bay
The Intra-Coastal Waterway (ICW) stretches up the east coast, from Miami in the south almost as far as New York in the north. This sheltered passage enables many small craft to make the 1600km (1000 miles) journey at any time of the year, without leaving the protection of the waterway.

It is a fascinating trip, mostly made under power. Supplies, fuel and water are readily available and you can stop at a marina every night. It certainly is an alternative to the outside passage (along the Atlantic coast) where bad weather can be encountered.

A boat with a draft of about 1.8m (6ft) should make it through the Intra-Coastal but a check on depths will be worthwhile. You should also know the height of your mast, and be able to step it, as there are many lowish bridges along the way.

The ICW has sand shoals, salt marshes, tidal flats, meandering creeks, wetland and marshland systems, and many off-limits nature reserves (wildlife refuges). Carry a dinghy so you can navigate the shallow channels and creeks. A folding bicycle is useful if you want to explore away from the water.

Towns and villages along the way welcome visiting boats, but not all have full-service marinas with ablution facilities, so be prepared to stay on board. Remember, this is not the sea, and in summer insects can be a problem, so consider fine mesh screens for the hatches and companionway.

The ICW is used particularly by cruisers heading south in the fall (autumn) and returning north in the spring – so it is busy at these times.

Chesapeake Bay is the largest inlet on the Atlantic seaboard. About 320km (200 miles) long and up to 64km (40 miles) wide, with several big rivers flowing into it, you could easily spend an entire summer cruising just this one body of water.

From Chesapeake Bay, you can sail north to New York, where you have a choice of continuing up the coast to Maine, the home of traditional wooden boat-building, and on to Nova Scotia, or up the Hudson River, connecting with the locks and canals which will take you through to Lakes Eire or Ontario and the rest of the Great Lakes.

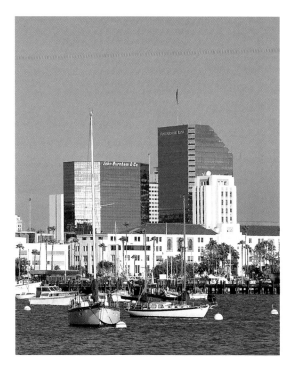

Florida Keys

The Florida Keys are a chain of around 800 islands stretching for 290km (180 miles) from the southeast tip of Florida. The northernmost island is Key Largo: the most southerly point, the Dry Tortugas, lies just 137km (85 miles) north of Havana.

Forty-two of the islands are linked by the Overseas Highway (US1), but most of them are accessible only by water. The keys form part of a huge coral reef that is protected by the Florida Keys National Marine Sanctuary, although game fishing, scuba diving and snorkelling are allowed.

Summers are hot and humid, but the winters are mild. Hurricane season is from August to October and storms are likely in late August and September.

There are many things to do in the Keys and it is worth making time to indulge in some nonsailing activities. In Key Largo, the Pilot House Marina offers a secluded anchorage close to the town centre. Scuba divers can view the Christ of the Deep, a 3m (10ft) statue submerged in 8m (25ft) of water at the John Pennekamp Coral Reef State Park. Deep-sea anglers should head for Islamorada, a noted game fishing centre, where uninhabited Indian Key is accessible only by boat. Those looking for an animal encounter can swim with dolphins at the Dolphin Research Centre at Marathon, on Grassy Key.

The Lower Keys start south of Seven Mile Bridge, the world's longest segmental bridge. Key West, at the end of the road (for landlubbers) is laid-back, with a lively nightlife centred around Duval Street and Mallory Square. Cruisers wanting to be part of the action should head for the Historic Seaport at the Key West Bight, just two blocks from Duval Street, or Pelican Landing Marina on Garrison Bight.

The cluster of seven islands that make up the Dry Tortugas National Park lie almost 113km (70 miles) south of Key West. Once an area of strategic military importance, it is now best known for its bird and marine life, as well as legends of pirate treasure.

Alternatively, from Palm Beach, you could make for the Bahamas, where there is excellent line-of-sight navigation, and the islands and cays are protected by one of the world's largest barrier reef systems.

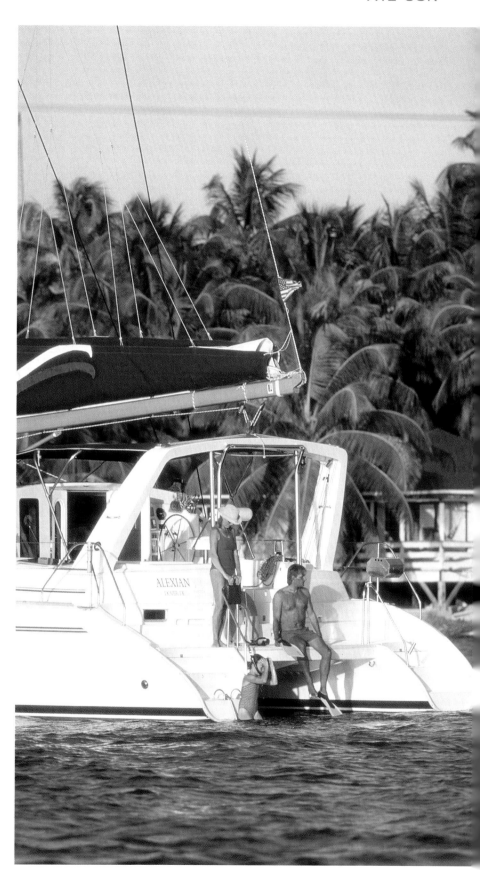

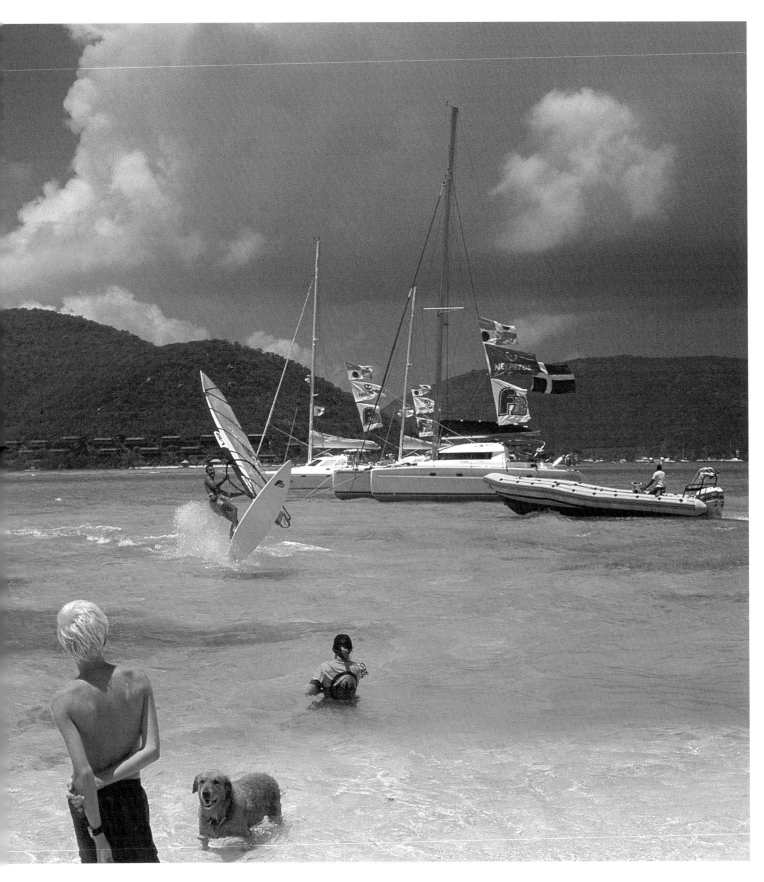

Hawaii

The seas surrounding the Hawaiian islands provide a challenge for the cruising sailor. It is not for nothing that some of the world's best surf is found on the reefs and shore breaks of these volcanic islands, which rise steeply from the depths of the Pacific.

The five main islands, Hawaii (or the Big Island), Maui, Oahu, Kauai and Molokai lie just south of the Tropic of Cancer, so there is plenty of sunshine and water temperatures average about 23°C (74°F) all year round, reaching highs of up to 27°C (80°F) in mid-summer.

For sailors the northeast trade winds are reliable, if fresh. Hawaiian weather patterns are affected by the surrounding warm seas as well as the high pressure zones in the north Pacific that bring cool, moist trade winds to the northeastern shores. Occasionally, however, the wind switches to the south or west, bringing stormy or very humid weather.

Wave action varies between islands and from winter to summer. Generally summer seas are gentle, but in winter, Pacific storms drive ocean swells towards the north shores, creating large waves. In areas such as South Point, off the Big Island, where the ocean floor rises from 1300 fathoms to breaking water in the space of a few kilometres, the combination of strong winds, huge waves and heavy seas can make sailing hazardous and cruising yachts are advised to keep well clear in these conditions.

In any event, most cruisers opt for the leeward shores, taking their time to marvel at the diversity of each of the islands: from Kilauea, the world's largest active volcano, spilling its lava into the sea off the Big Island, to the lush landscape of Kauai and the plunging cliffs and waterfalls of Maui.

Those wanting to get away from it all should head for Molokai, the least-developed of the islands, but if you are tired of solitude and seeking some action, then Oahu's beaches, particularly the famous Waikiki, will be more to your taste.

Oahu's leeward shore has extensive coral systems where visitors can experience supervised encounters with a wide variety of marine life, including whales, dolphins and turtles.

PANAMA CANAL

The 80km-long (50 miles) Panama Canal cuts through the narrow isthmus joining North and South America. It saves a 8000km (5000 miles) sail around Cape Horn and without it, many yachtsmen would never circumnavigate. It is possible to transit the Canal in a day, but most yachts spend a night at anchor in Gatun Lake.

Most yachts sail from the Caribbean to the Pacific. At Colón, the yacht is measured and fees paid (based on length; with up to 15m (50ft) LOA the lowest rate.)

At Gatun Locks, vessels are lifted 26m (85ft) in three steps to Gatun Lake, the highest point. After going through the 37km (23 miles) channel, the next stage is the Gaillard Cut, a spectacular gorge carved through sheer rock. Just 150m (498ft) wide in places, it was an amazing engineering feat when the Canal was built (1881–1914). After the San Pedro and Miraflores Locks, you sail under the Bridge of the Americas into the Pacific, your Panama Canal transit over.

You require an engine, four long warps (30m/100ft) able to hold three times boat's weight, four crew plus a helmsman, and plenty of fenders. First-timers should make the transit as a handler on another yacht before taking their own boat through. The Canal operates non-stop, 365 days a year. Yachts usually sail through the locks with large ships, so if your instructions are to be at a lock at two-thirty in the morning – be there!

Opposite *Storm clouds and strengthening winds herald the arrival of bad weather off Hawaii.*

Below *The gates of the Miraflores Lock are extremely high because of the tidal variation in the Pacific Ocean.*

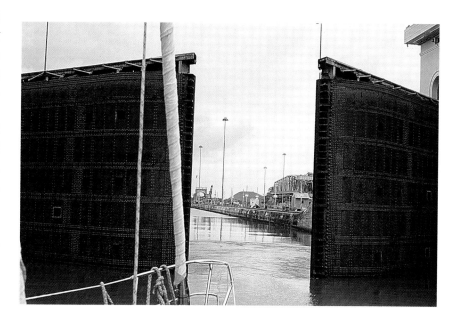

PACIFIC OCEAN

The Pacific covers an area about 15 times the size of the USA. It is the world's deepest ocean, averaging 4100m (13,800ft), with the Mariana Trench reaching nearly 11,000m (36,000ft) below sea level.

South of the equator, southeast trades blow and a cool current runs counter-clockwise, while northeast trades blow in the north, where there is a warm clock-wise gyre (circular system of currents). The winds meet in the inter-tropical convergence zone (also called the doldrums), an area of light, variable, squally weather. Tropical cyclones form in the summer months (as typhoons in Southeast Asia and hurricanes in Central America). The cyclical El Niño/La Niña phenomenon that occurs off the coast of South America influences weather in the western Pacific – indeed, in the entire western hemisphere.

Below *At anchor inside a sheltered Tahitian lagoon. Navigating the reefs around the islands is easy, as there are well-marked channels.*

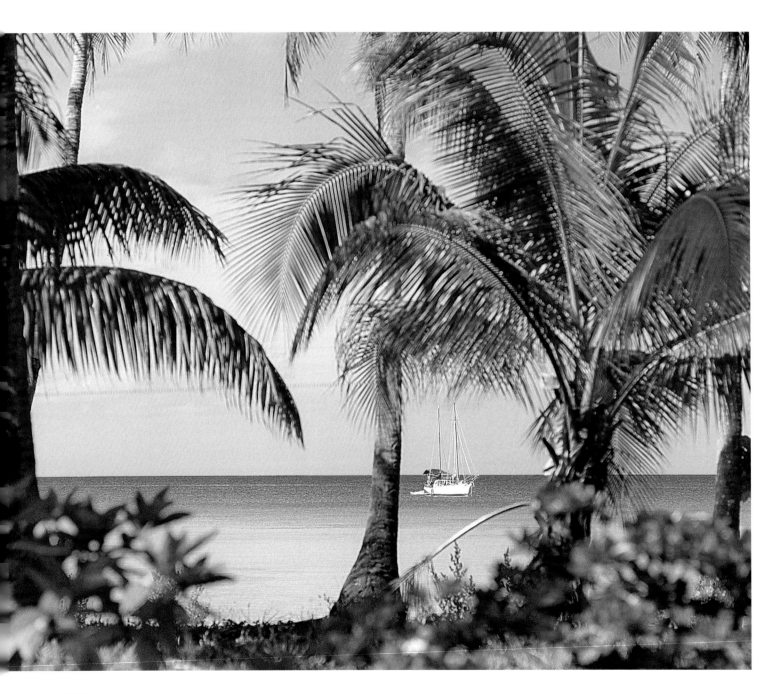

South Pacific (Tahiti, Fiji and Tonga)

From the Panama Canal, most sailors head for the islands of the South Pacific. This popular area is well supported by charter companies, which have bases on various island groups, and visiting yachts are assured of a warm welcome.

The beauty of the South Pacific is legendary, with coral atolls encircling aquamarine lagoons, and palm-fringed beaches giving way to tropical jungle pierced by weathered rocky outcrops.

The tropical weather is warm throughout the year with little temperature difference between summer and winter. As a general rule, the dry months (April to November), are the best for cruising, with dependable winds and temperatures above the 20°C (70°F) mark.

Within the island groups, much of the sailing is line of sight, but sailing between the islands requires open ocean skills. Sailing at night is discouraged because of the proliferation of coral reefs, and the large easterly compass deviation.

Sailing westward, one reaches French Polynesia, comprising the Society Islands (Tahiti, Mooréa, Bora Bora, Tahaa, Raiatéa and Huahine), the Marquises, and numerous smaller islands and islets.

One of the most popular destinations in the Society Islands is Bora Bora, a picture-perfect rendition of a typical South Sea island, with twin-peaked mountains, Otemanu and Pahia, that rise out of the sea as you approach. The passage to Bora Bora involves negotiating a difficult break in the barrier reef. Most channels between the reefs and the islands are well marked with cardinal and channel markers, but good charts and pilots are essential in these waters as the currents can be fast and swells heavy. Anchorages range from very deep to quite shallow.

Water and fresh provisions are available from local villages as well as the charter bases. Some hotels have private jetties, but the cost of moorings and services, including water, varies and sailing in these islands is generally expensive.

Tonga is slightly further south and the climate here is a bit cooler and less humid. Southeast trades ranging from 10–25 knots can be expected from May to September, with lighter breezes in summer.

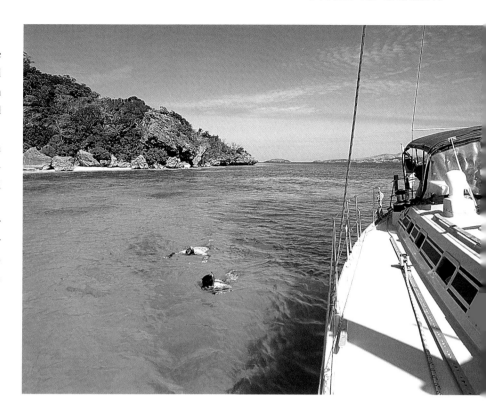

With 64 islands making up the Kingdom of Tonga, the 'friendly islands', there is plenty of good sailing, from open ocean crossings to sailing in the vicinity of the various islands, where distances are short and most sailing is line of sight. Anchorage is within the lee of the islands or reefs, while passages between islands are made in deep water.

At Mariner's Cave on Nuapapapu Island, a quick dive takes you through the underwater entrance, surfacing into a chamber filled with an eerie green mist and light streaming in from above; or you could take a dinghy into Swallow's Cave on Kapa Island. Attending a traditional Tongan feast is an essential part of any South Pacific cruise, although nowadays it is somewhat geared at the tourists.

Sailing in Fiji is complex, as the reef and coral system is extensive and not always well-charted. Local navigators are available and are to be recommended. Strong winds often come up later in the day, so it is sensible to find a good anchorage by mid-afternoon.

In all the South Pacific islands, take care to monitor the weather reports throughout summer, as many yachts have been lost to cyclones.

Above *Small islets dot the lagoons around Fiji, where the crystal clear waters and vibrant coral reefs invite exploration with a mask and snorkel .*

Opposite *A secluded anchorage on Hamilton Island, in the Whitsundays, part of the Great Barrier Reef.*

AUSTRALIA

Australia is bounded by the Indian Ocean, the Tasman Sea and the Pacific Ocean. Cape York and the Gulf of Carpentaria swelter in tropical heat, while Tasmania, lying between 40° and 45° south, is well in range of the cold winds that sweep across the Southern Atlantic. Tropical cyclones occur in the northeast between January and March. Generally, the best time for sailing is summer, between September and March.

The main sailing centres are the key coastal cities of Perth, Adelaide, Melbourne, Sydney and Hobart, while Brisbane and Cairns are important departure points for the Great Barrier Reef.

Below *Sydney has the world's largest natural harbour with 160km (100 miles) of shoreline to explore.*

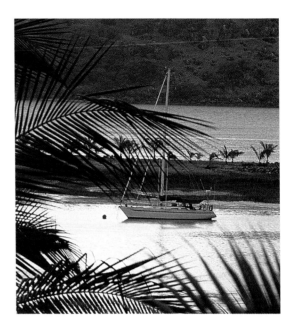

Great Barrier Reef

Covering an area of 260,000km^2 (100,400 sq miles), the Great Barrier Reef is made up of individual reefs and coral islands stretching 2000km (1200 miles) from Papua New Guinea to Lady Elliot Island, north of Brisbane. Although much of the reef barely rises above the surface of the water at low tide, it reaches a maximum depth of about 60m (200ft) at the southern end, where it nears the continental shelf.

The Whitsundays, a group of 74 islands in the Great Barrier Reef Marine Park, are ideal for cruising, with gentle southeast trades and short passages. Discover Whitehaven Beach, the deep gorge at Nara Inlet and a wide choice of swimming and snorkelling sites.

From Shute Harbour, on the mainland, day cruises depart for the Outer Reef Platform, a permanent structure on Hardy Reef where an underwater observatory and a small semi-submersible vessel enable even non-diving visitors to view the reef.

A wide range of sailing charters can be arranged from the towns of Gladstone, Mackay, Townsville and Cairns. Good charts and pilot books are essential for sailing anywhere in this area.

Responsible sailors try to avoid coral when anchoring or sailing in shallow waters, and it is best to sail by day only, finding a sheltered anchorage or making for a harbour or marina at night.

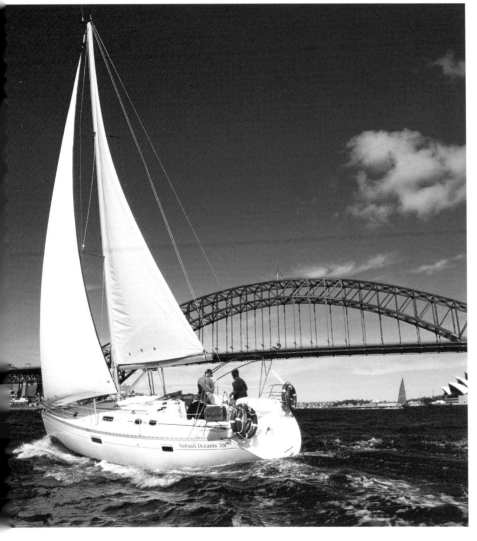

NEW ZEALAND

Extending through about 15 degrees of latitude, New Zealand is a land of contrasts; central North Island has a volcanic core, while the southeast has fjords to rival those of Norway. North Cape is about the same latitude as Sydney, while Stewart Island, off the southern tip, is situated deep in the Roaring Forties (only brave yachties choose to sail this tempestuous coast!).

The challenge of mastering the surrounding waters has turned New Zealanders into some of the world's top competitive sailors, but it is the sheer beauty of the coastline that attracts most cruisers.

The main centres of sailing activity are Auckland and Wellington on the North Island and Christchurch on the South Island, although most small coastal towns have some sort of harbour or marina.

Sailing in Auckland centres on Waitemata Harbour, which is sheltered by the islands of the Hauraki Gulf. From the city, one can sail to the Little and Great Barrier Islands and Coromandel Peninsula, or head north for the well-known Bay of Islands, where 86 islands and hundreds of kilometres of inlets provide an extensive and popular cruising ground.

The best time for sailing is from December to April, when the summer temperatures average 28°C (86°F) and the breezes are light, or during the spring, from September to November. From May to August, the winter winds are brisk and the temperatures are lower (around 20°C/69°F in June and July).

Russell, the main town in the Bay of Islands area, is on a narrow peninsula facing a sheltered bay that provides a good anchorage. Other options are the towns of Paihia and Opua (which has a charter base), or the protected harbour at Whangaroa.

South of Auckland, on the east coast, is the Bay of Plenty, a region blessed with a mild sunny climate. Take a break from the open ocean by heading for the inner harbour at Tauranga, which is situated within a protected bay. White Island, a still-active volcano in the bay, is an interesting side-trip, provided you don't get too close.

Gisborne, in Poverty Bay on the east coast, has a strong nautical heritage. It is a centre for big-game

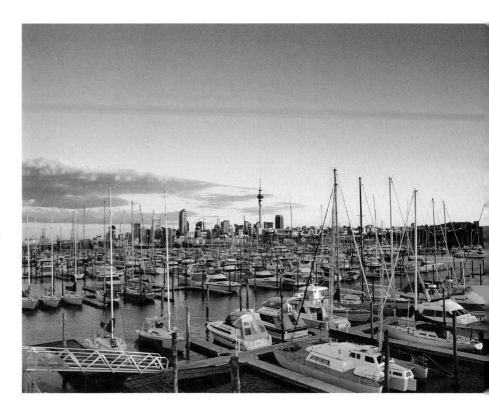

fishing. Situated at the southern tip of the North Island, Wellington has an extensive waterfront, where you will find marinas and plenty of facilities.

Across the Cook Strait are the deep, sheltered inlets of the Marlborough Sounds, where houses cling to forested slopes and boats are often a better means of transport than cars.

The Banks Peninsula juts out into the Pacific about halfway down the east coast. Here, the very English city of Christchurch shelters in the lee, while Akaroa Harbour, the sea-drowned valley of an extinct volcano, forms a deep natural bay surrounded by rolling hills and pasture that reaches to the water's edge.

The water is colder here, and the temperatures are lower, even in summer, as you head for the southern town of Dunedin.

In summer, many cruisers head for the fjords that cut into the lower western end of the South Island. Here deep sounds, such as Doubtful, George and Milford, are havens of beauty, reflecting the snow-covered peaks in their tranquil waters. There are few towns in this area, making good sailing skills and a well-equipped boat a necessity.

Above *Westhaven Marina in Auckland: the city was home to the 2003 America's Cup, which Team New Zealand lost to the Swiss challenger,* Alinghi.

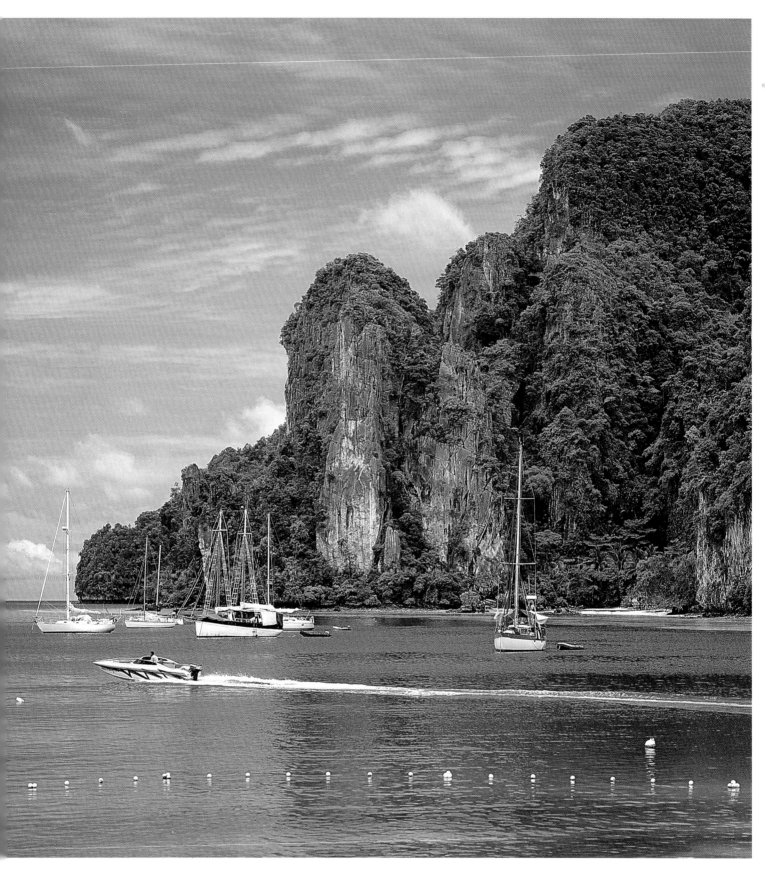

INDIAN OCEAN

The round-the-world route via the trade winds takes us from northern Australia via the Cocos Keeling Islands to Mauritius and on to South Africa, or via the Chagos Islands and the Seychelles, up the Red Sea, through the Suez Canal and into the Mediterranean.

The transocean passage to Mauritius offers excellent trade wind sailing. Good stopping points along the way include Christmas Island, Cocos Keeling Islands, Rodrigues, Réunion and Madagascar.

To make a west-east passage, go to about latitude 38° south from Cape Town or Durban, where you get the Westerlies without the gales of the Roaring Forties, and sail across to Fremantle in Western Australia. From there you can decide what to do in the knowledge that you can get weather forecasts and there are ports in which you can take shelter.

Thailand

Warm turquoise water, palm-fringed beaches, sheer limestone cliffs, spectacular scenery and the fragrant allure of Thai food, make Thailand a popular stop-over for sailors cruising the South China Sea. Chartering is well-established here and it is an ideal place to combine an exotic holiday with excellent sailing.

Phuket, on the Andaman Sea, has long been a favoured destination for visitors from the West. Phuket Yacht Club, in the south of the island, has good moorings, a comfortable hotel and an annual regatta, the King's Cup, which attracts sailors from all over the world. The regatta has classes for everyone, from non-spinnaker cruising boats to sleek racing craft taking each other on in the overnight race to a nearby *koh*, or island. The regatta is held in December, when the north-east monsoon winds are blowing steadily.

At Laem Phrao Bay, in northeastern Phuket, the Yacht Haven Marina offers a full range of services and can accomodate boats of all sizes. It is a gateway to Phang Nga Bay, where a well-visited destination is Koh Tapoo, the island made famous in the James Bond movie *Goldfinger*, as well as the Phi Phi islands and the many secluded anchorages around Krabi. Those who prefer to get away from it all head for the

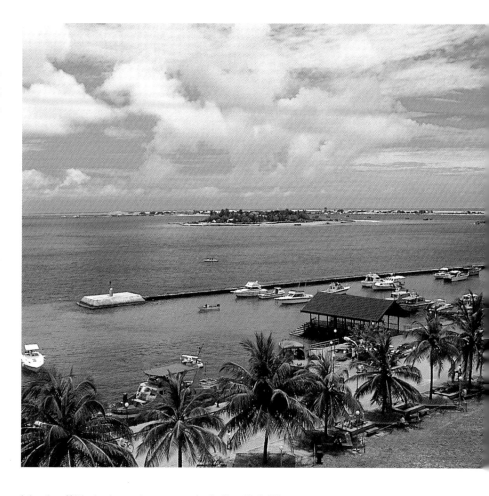

islands off Phuket's southern coast, including Koh Hi, Koh Mai Thon and Yai Bay. Ocean crossings can be made to the Andaman and Nicobar islands, which belong to India.

Maldives

The Maldives Archipelago lies south of India and just north of the equator. It comprises 26 atolls, made up of about 1200 small islands, the majority of which are uninhabited. It is coral, not rock, that forms the substructure of these low-lying islands which look as if they could disappear beneath the sea at any moment. (In all seriousness, a small rise in the water level due to global warming or other quirks of nature, could wipe out much of the Maldives.)

The coral reefs around the islands are considered to be some of the world's best, and form the basis of the economy, drawing thousands of divers every year to the country's resorts.

Above *The inner harbour at Male, the main island in the Maldives Archipelago.*

Opposite *Sheer limestone cliffs plunging into the sea, such as here at Tonsai Bay, are typical of Thailand.*

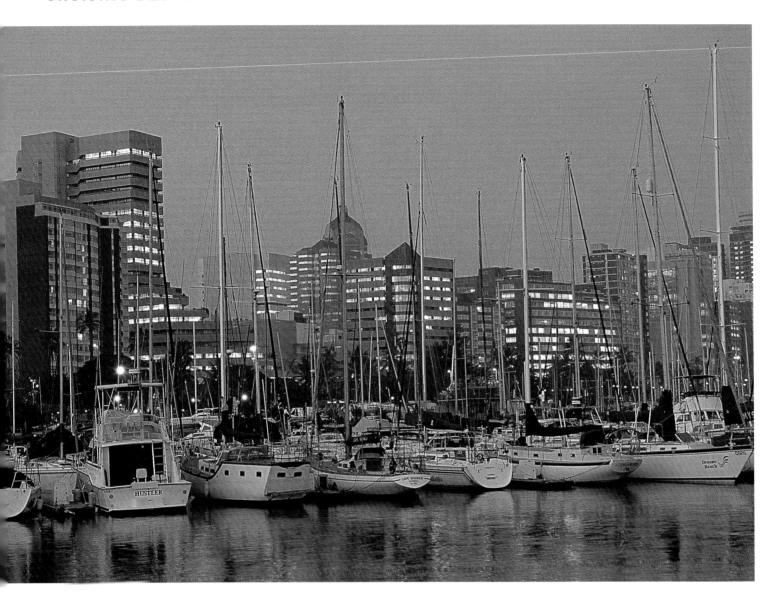

Above *As dusk falls, Durban's city lights illuminate boats in the small craft harbour on the city's Victoria Embankment.*

SOUTH AFRICA

Most yachts heading across the Indian Ocean to South Africa stop at Mauritius before setting course for Richards Bay or Durban. A cyclone belt forms east of Madagascar from January to June, so it is advisable to be in South Africa by late December or early January.

The eastern coast of South Africa has a bad reputation among yachtsmen, mainly because of the giant waves encountered when southwesterly gales blow against the Agulhas Current. Careful monitoring of the weather should enable you to avoid such blows but, if you do encounter them, ignore the old adage that you need sea room! Come close into the coast (2km/1½ miles off the breakers) to avoid the giant waves that give shipping such a hard time (see also p66).

Heading south, you need to know all possible places to shelter from the southwesterly gales: East London is 260 nautical miles south of Durban, then comes Port Elizabeth, Port St Francis, Knysna, Mossel Bay and Struis Bay, before rounding Cape Agulhas, the southernmost tip of Africa. The headland of Cape Point, also called the Cape of Good Hope, is a dramatic landmark en route to Cape Town.

If you are planning an Atlantic crossing, you should leave South Africa between January and March.

SAILING IN COLD WATERS

Unlike the popular trade wind routes, relatively few cruising boats travel the frigid waters of high latitudes (nearer to the poles) and you are likely to get a warm welcome in ports where the arrival of a foreign yacht is not an everyday occurrence.

In cold waters, it is important to constantly monitor weather forecasts for the surrounding area and for the direction you are travelling in, to get a picture of what systems to expect in the days ahead.

If gale force winds or snow storms are forecast, ensure both you and your boat are fully able to handle the expected conditions before you put to sea. Remember that wind-blown spray and heavy rain can reduce visibility, creating a dangerous situation if you are sailing close inshore or near shipping lanes.

Popular high latitude destinations include north-eastern USA and Canada, including the Great Lakes, and the northwest coast of Canada and the Gulf of Alaska. In Europe, the Baltic Sea and Scandinavian coast offer a combination of sheltered fjords and open ocean passages.

In the southern hemisphere, yachts visiting the Falkland Islands, or making the notorious passage around Cape Horn will encounter testing weather conditions, as will boats sailing around the tip of New Zealand's South Island. The infamous Roaring Forties tend to be the domain of round-the-world racers rather than cruising yachties.

Below *Cold water sailing demands an investment in heavy weather clothing that is not necessary in the tropics.*

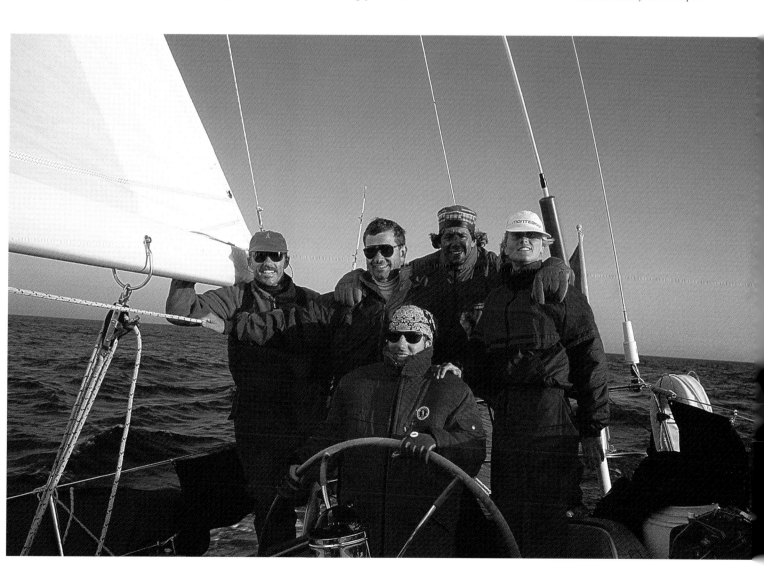

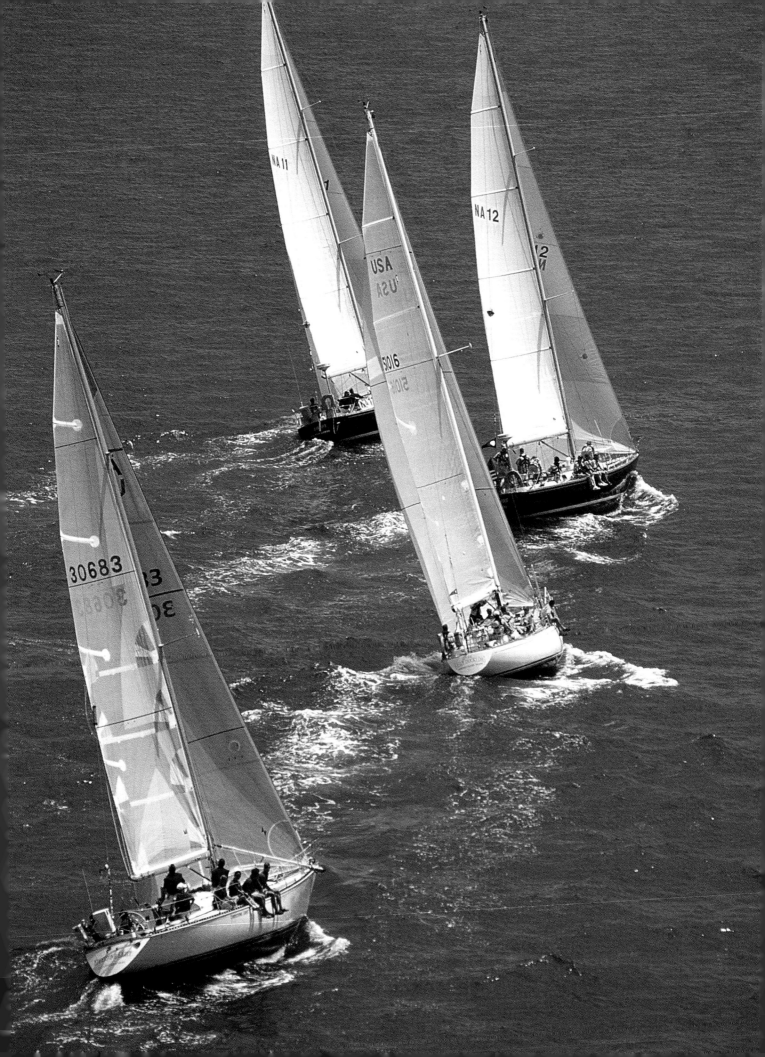

RACING

Today, top yacht racing at international levels is almost exclusively confined to professional sailors. However, many technological innovations developed for racing soon become the standard for cruising boats. This is true of materials such as the sophisticated laminates used in hi tech racing yachts. Even carbon fibre masts, which were permitted in the Volvo Race for the first time in 2001, are already appearing on cruising boats.

Events like the Volvo Round the World Race (formerly the Whitbread) are heavily dependent on sponsorship and extensive media coverage. Entrants spend several years training with full-time crews, who are paid good salaries. Boats are purpose-built for each specific race, using the most advanced design and technology available.

This level of racing has isolated the average yachtsman from participation in most international events but yacht clubs and sailing organizations continue to ensure that various long-distance races remain accessible to smaller yachts which are capable of both racing and cruising. These range from day and overnight races in local waters to ocean crossings. While competition between individual yachts in the same class might be fierce, the events are usually open to boats from a number of different classes all competing on handicap.

Opposite *The Class II start in the 1998 Newport Bermuda race. This classic offshore event attracts cruiser racers as well as top-level ocean racing yachts.*

Racing in a cruising boat

Racing is a far cry from cruising in terms of a boat's capabilities, crew skills and training, the calibre of the sails and other equipment, the standard of navigation required and many other factors.

If you want to become really involved in racing, you must weigh up various factors, including whether you can afford it and whether you have the time and energy to train a crew and keep them together. Can your family life and business commitments survive the dedication that competitive racing demands?

If the answer to these questions is no, then stick to cruising or opt for fun races – there are enough events around the world to satisfy all but the most single-minded sailor.

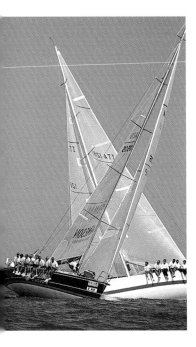

Above *Successful racing requires crew members who are able to dedicate regular time to practising.*

Cruising rallies
The annual Atlantic Rally for Cruisers (ARC), a 2700-nautical mile (4344km) event, is sailed from Las Palmas, Canary Islands, to St Lucia, Lesser Antilles. Starting in November, the passage on the northeast trades takes 12 to 24 days.

The largest transoceanic sailing event in the world, it attracts over 150 entries each year, in a number of classes. The ARC is open to cruising monohulls from 27ft (8m) LOA (length overall) and catamarans ranging from 25–60ft (7–18m) LOA, sailed by a minimum crew of two.

The World Cruising handicap is used to calculate the results in the cruising classes, in which motoring is permitted. More competitive boats can compete in a racing class under the IRC system, held under the auspices of the RORC (Royal Ocean Racing Club).

The ARC is ideal for sailors who are crossing an ocean for the first time, or those who prefer to transit under controlled conditions and in radio contact with other yachts in the fleet. By simply complying with the event's safety regulations, novices can learn a tremendous amount about the ocean-crossing game.

Despite cruising races like the ARC or Cape to Rio appearing to offer a 'safe' way to cross the ocean, all blue water passages carry an element of risk. In the 2002 ARC, a man-overboard (MOB) situation resulted

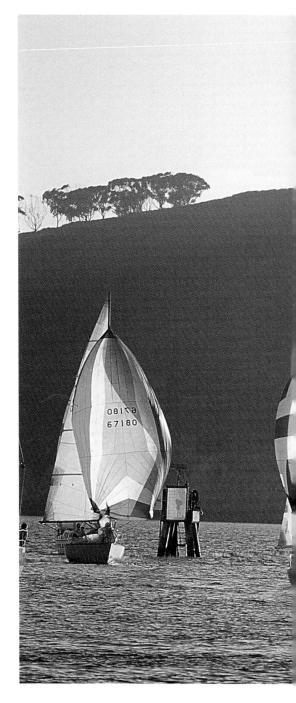

in a tragic death, while another cruiser participating in the race was abandoned and scuttled after its rudder broke in heavy seas and a jury rudder subsequently failed. In both instances, help was forthcoming from the fleet, but the loss of life and the emotional cost to those involved in both situations are testimony to the unpredictability of the sea.

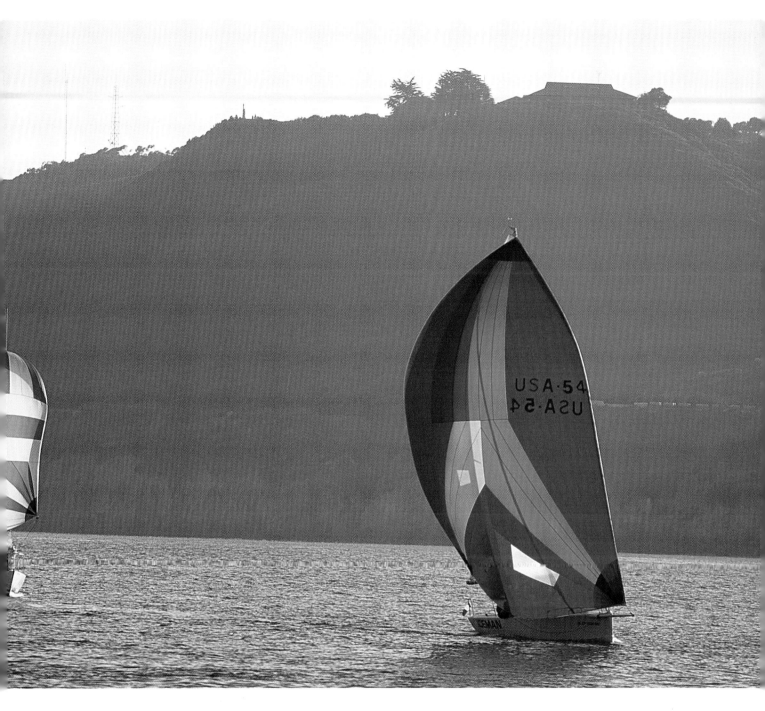

Class rallies

A camaraderie, even a friendly rivalry, often develops between the owners of certain types of boats.

An example of what can be put together is demonstrated by Oyster, a UK company which makes a series of well-finished pilot-house cruisers whose satisfied, and loyal, owners ensure there are always a number of Oysters on the oceans of the world. An Oyster class rally held in Antigua was remarkable for the number of these boats that made the passage to the Caribbean just to attend the rally, as well as for the level of competition between the respective owners. Evenings were 'party time' and the result was a thoroughly enjoyable week.

Above *Smaller cruising yachts competing in class rallies off San Diego.*

131

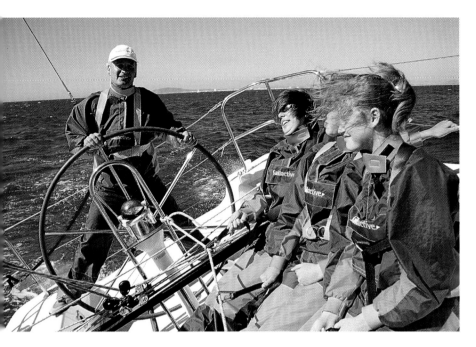

Weekend racing is usually taken seriously, requiring a well-trained crew capable of tacking fast and often, with spinnakers frequently used. The course is often long, and navigation may be required to locate the marks. In constrast, mid-week racing is much more relaxed. The course is short and straightforward and most skippers use regular sails, rather than racing sails. Spinnakers are generally excluded from the smaller classes. Non-sailors are welcome aboard and many new sailors have been introduced to the sport through an evening race. Social events are often held afterwards and the club pub is usually well-patronized.

Club racing is usually covered by a yacht's comprehensive insurance policy, so owners do not have to face the extra expense of a 'racing risks' policy.

Above *Club racing provides an ideal opportunity to train novice sailors.*

Opposite *In light following winds, spinnakers will catch any hint of a breeze that might enable you to get ahead of a competitor, such as in this club race off San Diego.*

Owner's associations

There are many national and international associations of owners of a particular make or class of boat which do a great job of keeping owners in touch with the activities of their class.

The 8.5m (28ft) Albin Vega is a case in point. Hundreds of these light-displacement vessels were built in Sweden during the late 1960s and 1970s. They are now found all over the world and are sought out by those who want to make long passages safely on a low budget. A newsletter keeps members informed of activities, rallies, low-key competitive events and cruises. The loyalty to this little boat, which hasn't been built for years, is quite incredible.

Club racing

Yacht clubs around the world hold regular races, using their local PHRF handicap system, where boats race against similar models in clearly-defined classes. Starts are often staggered so that smaller craft do not get in the way of the bigger boats, allowing cruisers to participate alongside racing yachts. The fleet may also be split into spinnaker and non-spinnaker classes.

Races may be one-offs or form part of a series that lasts all season. Whether one takes the results seriously is up to the individual skipper and crew.

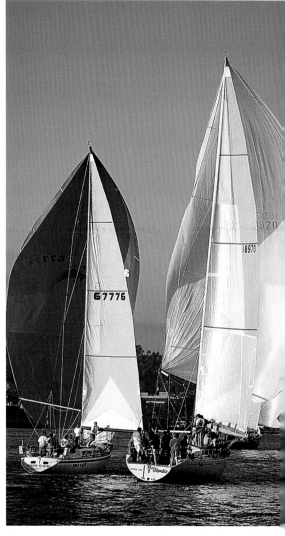

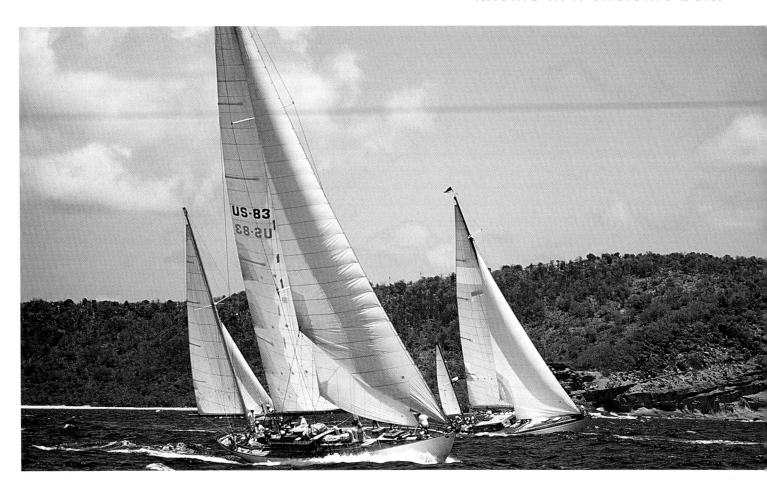

Regattas

Many well-established week-long regattas cater for the average cruiser racer, with classes for smaller boats or local 'one design' yachts as well as races for professionally crewed hi tech racing boats.

There are too many regattas to list them all, but some well-known ones include Cowes Week, the USA's Block Island Regatta and San Francisco Big Boat Regatta, the Swan Worlds, which are usually held in Sardinia, and Ireland's Cork Week.

Probably the most famous regatta is Cowes Week, which is held annually in August under the auspices of the various yacht clubs based in Cowes (see also the Fastnet Race on p134).

Cowes, a town on the Isle of Wight in the English Channel, is often considered to be the home of sailing, and this is a fantastic regatta indeed. Not only do the top classes of hi tech yachts, crewed by professionals, compete for honours, but many handicap classes for cruisers and local One Designs also exist. One of the biggest classes racing every year is the X-Class One Design, where some of the boats are over 70 years old, yet the competition is fierce. One of the highlights is the Round the Island race, a 50-nautical-mile course sailed anticlockwise around the Isle of Wight. There is something for everyone at Cowes.

The Swan Regatta started out as a small event run for owners of the various Swans built by Nautor, and has now been built up into an important regatta.

Many Caribbean nations hold annual race weeks. Most, such as Antigua Week, started off as low-key events, but they now attract a wide range of cruisers and racers. Some of the Caribbean races have created classes for classic yachts, which have gained a large following in recent years, particularly in the USA.

To sum things up, if you want to race your boat at any level, you should be able find a suitable event almost anywhere in the world.

Above *Antigua Race Week attracts yachts from all over the world, drawn as much by the racing as by the party spirit.*

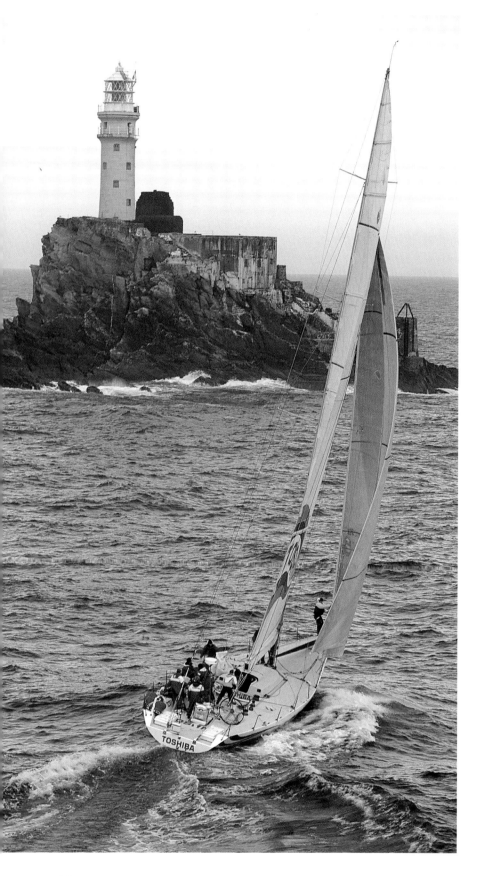

RACES OPEN TO CRUISING BOATS

The Fastnet Race

Perhaps the best-known long-distance race in the world is the UK's Fastnet Race, which takes place every second year (uneven years) at the end of Cowes Week (early August). The course takes boats from Cowes around the southern tip of England to the Fastnet Rock, which is rounded to port, and back to the finish line off Plymouth, a distance of 608 nautical miles.

This is a challenging, tactical race, with big tides and variable weather to contend with, but it remains a goal for many seasoned sailors.

It is sailed under the auspices of the Royal Ocean Racing Club, the Royal Yacht Squadron and the Royal Western Yacht Club of Plymouth, in association with FICO (Fédération Internationale de la Course Océanique). Classes include IRC (for yachts up to 30m/100ft LOA), IRM, multihulls, a two-handed division and IMS/ORC club classes for a minimum of 15 entries.

A new speed record was set in 1999 by the 60ft multihull *Sayonara*, which reached a top speed of 15.98 knots. France's Catherine Chabaud holds the record for the fastest time to complete the race. In 1999, sailing her Open 60 *Whirlpool-Europe 2*, she took five days, 22 hours and 59 minutes. The 2001 race was won by the French multihull *Eure et Loire* in a fantastically fast time of one day, 18 hours and 19 minutes, reaching speeds of 25 knots on both the outward and return legs.

In 1979 the Fastnet fleet was decimated by a severe gale. Nineteen lives were lost and many boats were abandoned or seriously damaged by being rolled over. The incident focused attention on the stability factor, as a subsequent investigation found that, in order to make racing yachts rate better under the IOR (International Offshore Rule), they were being made less and less stable.

Furthermore, many of the abandoned boats were found afloat days later, leading to conclusions that it is better to stay with your boat than take to the life raft, unless your yacht is about to sink under you.

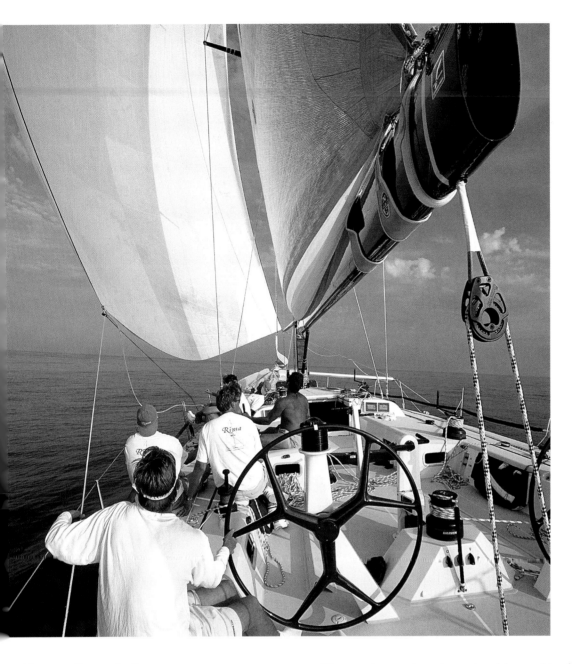

Left *The Farr 60 maxi* Rima, *owned by Isam Kabbami, finished fourth in its class in the 1998 Newport Bermuda Race, with an elapsed time of 100 hours, 32 minutes, 42 seconds.*

Opposite Toshiba, *a Whitbread 60, rounding Fastnet Rock during the 1997 Fastnet Race, which was won by the German maxi* Morning Glory, *skippered by Hasso Plattner.*

Newport Bermuda Race

Sponsored jointly by the Cruising Club of America (CCA) and the Royal Bermuda Yacht Club, this biennial race (sailed in even years) covers a distance of 635 nautical miles (1022km) from Newport, Rhode Island, to St David's Head, Bermuda.

It is a hotly contended, tactical race that tests seamanship with a course that crosses the fast-flowing, unpredictable Gulf Stream. Boats that accurately anticipate its meanders usually do well on handicap.

The race is open to racing and cruising yachts of not less than 8.4m (27.5ft) with a valid IMS or Americap rating certificate, sailed by a minimum of four crew (except for double-handed entries), in both spinnaker and non-spinnaker classes.

The Newport Bermuda Race was first held in 1906 and took place on an annual basis until 1926 when it began alternating with the Fastnet Race. In 1996, George Coumantaros' *Boomerang* set an elapsed time record of 57 hours, averaging just over 11 knots.

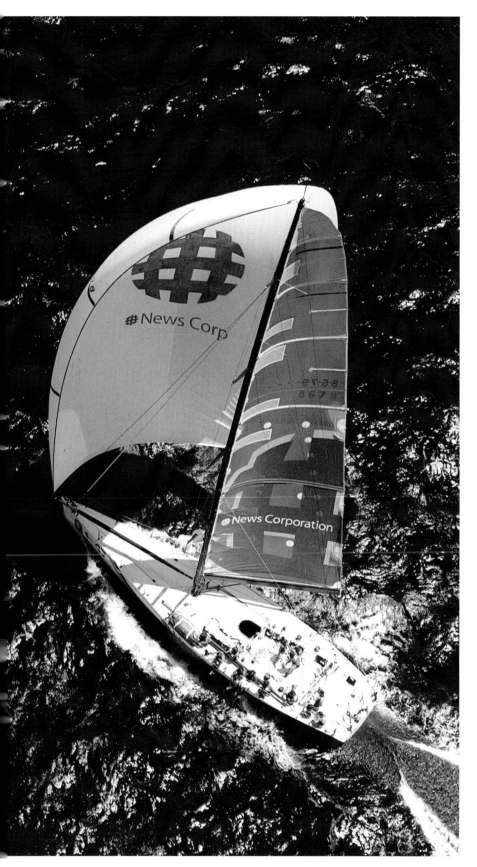

Sydney Hobart Race

This classic offshore race, which always starts on 26 December, takes the fleet in a southerly direction across the Bass Straight and down the Tasmanian coast to Hobart. It is 630 nautical miles long (1013km) and is usually very tough. The fleet often meets strong southwesterly head winds, which blow against the current in fairly shallow water, giving rise to mountainous seas and resulting in many participants not finishing because of the conditions.

There are divisions for boats that hold an IRC Certificate, an inexpensive document issued by the UK's RORC (Royal Ocean Racing Club). It is based on a very simple rule and caters for the private boat owner who wants to compete at his own level.

In 1998 the race was hit by a storm which resulted in the loss of six lives and caused untold damage. Like the Fastnet disaster some 20 years earlier, an enquiry led to the already-strict Offshore Racing requirements being tightened up even further.

The overall winner of the 2002 race was Sydney yachtsman Bob Steele, sailing the 46ft *Quest*, after a nail-biting finish by *Zeus II*, which came within four minutes of claiming the coveted Tattersall's Trophy.

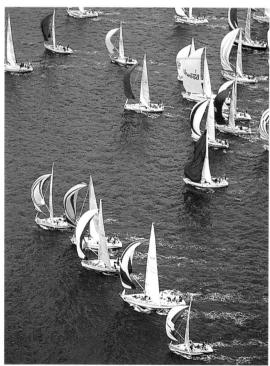

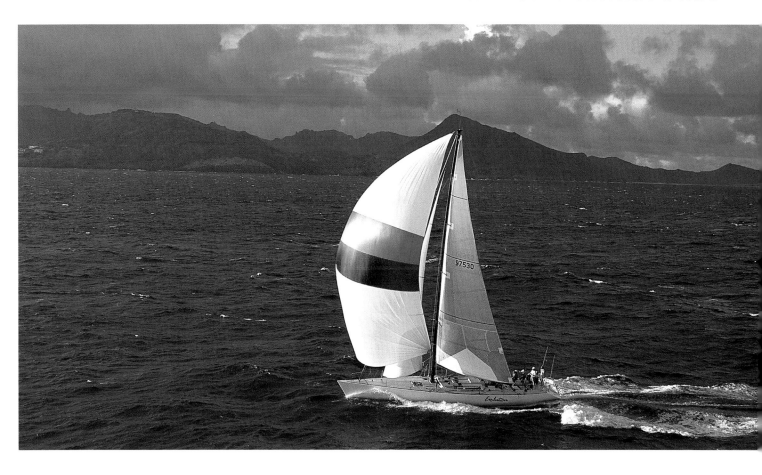

Transpac Race

The Transpacific Race is run biennially from Los Angeles to Hawaii under the auspices of the Transpacific Yacht Club (the last race was July 2003).

The 2225-nautical-mile (3500km) race starts near Point Fermin, California, leaves Santa Catalina Island to port and ends off Diamond Head, Oahu. The winning boats cover the distance in eight to 10 days.

A predominantly downwind race, it prompted the development of 'downwind sleds', light-displacement maxi boats with plenty of sail that are optimized for high-speed sailing, and have found a particular home on the US west coast.

The race is open to monohull and multihull classes with IMS or Americap II certificates or a Southern California PHRF rating as applicable for special classes. Monohulls must be at least 30ft (9m) LOA and multihulls at least 45ft (14m) LOA.

Staggered starts, some days apart, cater for the needs of slower cruising yachts, such as the Cal 40s, traditional 40ft (12m) fibreglass sloops which took line honours a number of times in the 1960s and which still have a dedicated band of enthusiasts keen to re-establish the class.

Other classes include those for older and heavier displacement boats, double-handed entries and multihulls. Racing is within a division or class, as well as against the fleet overall, with time adjusted according to handicap.

One of the key factors of this race is the position of the Pacific high, an area of calms which must be avoided by race-winning boats. The return sail is often a hard slog against head winds (something often left to delivery crews, as weary competitors fly home after a stint of four hours on, four hours off shifts for the duration of the race).

This downwind event was first sailed in 1906 and is now one of the longest-standing ocean races. (The America's Cup, which was first held in 1851, has the distinction of being the world's oldest yacht race.)

Above *Brack Duker's Santa Cruz 70,* Evolution, *in the 1995 Transpac Race. Designed for downwind sailing, the boat can achieve tremendous speeds with the spinnaker up.*

Opposite left *The Volvo 60* News Corp *in action, with an asymmetrical spinnaker set.*

Opposite right *A colourful spinnaker start to the 1994 Sydney Hobart race.*

Cape to Rio Race

This 5695km (3540 miles) transatlantic race takes place every three years, the most recent event being in January 2003. It is a joint venture between South African Sailing, Cape Town's Royal Cape Yacht Club (RCYC), and Iate Clube do Rio de Janeiro.

While competition in the racing classes is intense, there is also a cruising division, which starts a week earlier. Many South African cruisers use the Rio race as the first leg of a longer voyage, taking advantage of daily radio reports and assistance with port clearance in both Cape Town and Rio de Janeiro.

An important factor in this downwind race is the South Atlantic high, an area of calm winds directly between Cape Town and Rio de Janeiro. The island of Trindade serves as a mark on the course (boats have to pass to the north), but instead of taking the rhumb line (direct course) from Cape Town to Trindade, the fleet has to go to about 20° south to avoid the high.

As the fleet nears South America, local conditions exert their influence and racing becomes more tactical as skippers try to judge the winds and weather.

Line honours in the first race (1971) went to UK skippers Robin Knox-Johnston and Leslie Williams in the 72ft ketch *Ocean Spirit*, which made the crossing in 23 days at an average speed of 6.7 knots. The course record was set in 2000 by the 75ft *Zephyrus IV*, in 12 days, 16 hours, 49 minutes – an indication of the technological changes in boat design over the last 30 years.

Light winds slowed the fleet in the 2003 event. Line honours in the monohull class went to the 81ft (25m) maxi *Morning Glory*, which finished in 16 days, 8 hours, 31 minutes, while the overall winner on handicap was the 42ft (13m) *Baleka*.

Below and opposite *The 2003 Cape to Rio race started in ideal conditions. Twelve days later, the Swedish trimaran* Nicator *crossed the line at Rio in an elapsed time of 12 days, 23 hours, 47 minutes.*

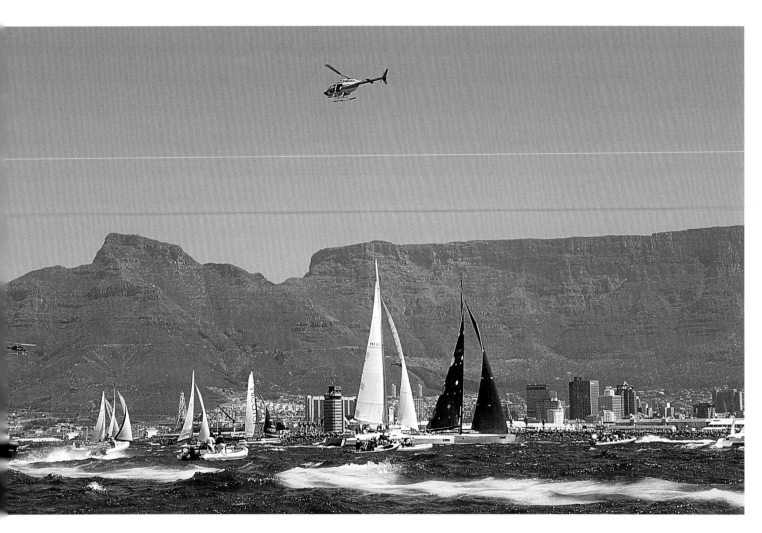

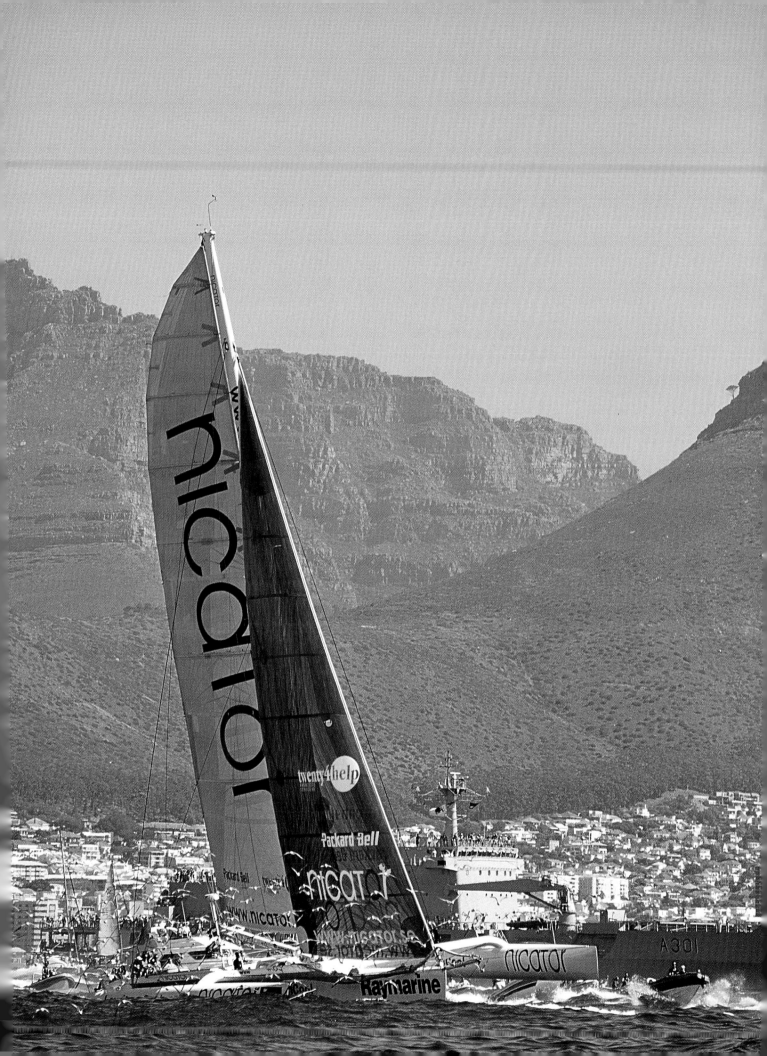

Aft At or near the stern of a vessel. (See also Forward.)

Ahull A sailboat is laying ahull when it is lying with all sails furled; associated with riding out gales.

Anchor rode The anchor line, rope or cable connecting the anchor to the vessel.

Apparent wind The direction of wind over the deck, calculated as the speed and direction of true wind plus the speed and direction of the boat. (See True wind.)

Astern Behind. To go astern means to reverse.

Beam The maximum width of a boat.

Bear away To alter course away from the wind.

Bearing An object's direction, expressed in compass degrees. Bearings can be true or magnetic.

Beating Sailing to windward (upwind), by tacking.

Bight A curved or looped section of a rope. Also an indentation in a coastline.

Bitter end The end of a warp (rope) or chain.

Boom A spar, or pole. The foot of the mainsail is normally attached to a boom.

Bosun's chair A seat made of strong fabric or wood, used to hoist a person up the mast in safety.

Bow The forward section of a vessel.

Broach To slew in a following sea or wind. The boat rounds up violently and can heel to an alarming angle.

Broad reach A point of sail between a reach and a run.

Bulkhead A structural, normally watertight partition running across the width of a vessel.

Burgee A triangular flag, often representing the yacht club to which the vessel belongs.

Close-hauled A sailing vessel is close-hauled when sailing as close to the wind as possible.

Cockpit Area towards the stern of a yacht from which the helmsman steers and the crew trims the sails.

Companionway The main entrance into a sea-going sailboat, usually via a hatch leading to a ladder.

Dead reckoning (DR) A method of navigating by recording the course sailed, leeway, speed, current drift, etc at regular intervals, starting from a known position (see also Observed position).

Displacement The weight of water a vessel displaces when floating normally. The weight of the displaced water equals the weight of the boat.

Downwind A point of sailing with the wind aft of the beam; the term is used for broad reaching or running.

Draught/draft The depth of a vessel under the water, from the waterline to the lowest point of the keel.

Ebb tide The tide is ebbing when it flows back from high to low water. (See also Flood tide.)

Ensign A flag flown to indicate a vessel's nationality.

Fathom A unit of measure, normally used with regard to water depth. One fathom = 1.8m (6ft).

Fix A fix is the vessel's position taken by obtaining accurate bearings by compass, sextant or other means.

Flood tide The tide is flooding when it rises from low to high water. (See also Ebb tide.)

Forward ('forrard') Towards the bow of a vessel.

Free wind Wind is aft of the beam, or running free.

Gimbals A swivelling device which enables a galley stove or compass card to remain level.

Go about To turn a sailing vessel through the head-to-wind position in order to change tacks.

GPS Global positioning System, an instrument which fixes a craft's position by means of satellites.

Gunwale ('gunnel') The top edge of the hull where, in the case of a decked vessel, the hull meets the deck.

Gybe To change course by turning the stern through the wind. A fore-and-aft sail will be moved from the left side of the boat to the right, or vice versa.

Halyard A rope or wire used to hoist sails.

Heading The compass direction in which the vessel is pointed.

Headsail A triangular sail set forward of the mast.

Heads The vessel's toilet(s).

Head-to-wind Pointed directly into the wind.

Heave to To stop the boat, normally by sheeting a headsail to windward.

Heel To lean over or list.

Helm A wheel or tiller by which a vessel is steered.

Holding ground Ground into which an anchor can dig.

In irons A sailing vessel is 'in irons' when it is pointing directly into the wind and has lost its momentum.

Inshore Close to, or towards, the shore.

Isobars Lines on a weather map which join areas of equal barometric pressure.

Jury rig A temporary arrangement to replace damaged rigging and/or spars.

Knot Unit of speed. One knot equals a speed of one nautical mile per hour.

Lanyard A short length of line or rope for attaching items so they will not be lost overboard.

Lee The sheltered area downwind of a vessel (away from the direction from which the wind is blowing).

Leeward ('loo'ard') Towards the lee side; the direction to which the wind is blowing. (See also Windward.)

Life line A safety line fitted around the deck, or fore and aft, to prevent the crew from slipping overboard.

Log An instrument used to measure a boat's speed through water and distance travelled. Also a logbook.

Mainsail The principal sail of a sailboat, always aft of the main mast in a fore-and-aft rigged boat.

Mainsheet The rope, normally run through a series of blocks, that controls the trim of the mainsail.

Mark A fixed feature, either afloat or ashore, used as a guide for navigation.

Mayday A distress signal sent in a case of extreme emergency or when life is in danger.

Millibar Unit of barometric pressure used to measure atmospheric pressure (1000 millibars = 1 bar).

Nautical mile Unit of length equal to 1852m (6076ft). Also equal to one minute of latitude.

Observed position Position obtained by direct observation of features on a chart, or by observing celestial bodies by sextant. (See also Dead reckoning.)

Offshore At some distance from the shore.

Onshore On or towards land (e.g. an onshore breeze).

Painter A line used to tow or tie up a small boat.

Pilot A person qualified to navigate a vessel into or out of harbours or rivers; also a navigation reference.

Plot To mark a boat's position on a chart.

Port The left side of a vessel when facing the bow.

Port tack A yacht is on port tack when the wind comes over the port (left) side. (See also Starboard tack.)

Prow The front section of a vessel including the bow.

Pulpit A guard rail at the bow of a boat, usually built of stainless steel or aluminium tubing.

Pushpit A guard rail at the stern of a boat.

Race A rapid current, often caused by restricting the flow of water through a narrow channel.

Reach A point of sailing when the wind is approximately at right angles to the boat.

Reef To reduce the size (area) of a sail for operation in heavy weather.

Run To sail with the wind directly behind the centreline of the boat.

Running rigging The sheets and halyards which control the raising, lowering and set of the sails. (See also Standing rigging.)

Sea anchor A drogue-shaped anchor streamed in bad weather to slow the boat down.

Sheet The rope attached to the clew of a sail or, via a tackle, to the boom; it is used to control sail trim.

Spinnaker A large, normally lightly constructed, full headsail for downwind use; usually multicoloured.

Standing rigging The shrouds and stays that support the mast/s. (See also Running rigging.)

Stand on To maintain a course. A vessel with right-of-way is known as the stand-on vessel.

Starboard The right of a vessel when facing the bow.

Starboard tack A sailing vessel is said to be on starboard tack when the wind comes over the starboard, or right, side. (See also Port tack.)

Stern The aft section of a vessel.

Tack To turn a sailboat through the eye of the wind (to go from port tack to starboard tack and vice versa).

Trade wind A wind blowing obliquely towards the equator (from the northeast in the northern hemisphere, southeast in the south), between latitudes 30° N and S.

True wind Speed and direction of the actual wind as if the vessel is not moving. (See also Apparent wind.)

Upwind Sailing upwind of a vessel means sailing to windward of it. (See also Windward.)

UT Universal Time. Formerly GMT.

Veer A clockwise shift in wind direction ('back' is an anticlockwise shift in wind direction).

Warp A rope used to moor or secure a vessel.

Weather side The upwind, or windward, side of a boat.

Windward Direction from which the wind is blowing; the weather side of a boat. (See also Upwind.)

PHOTOGRAPHIC CREDITS

Copyright rests with the following photographers and/or their agents. All images not listed below are by Neil Corder for NHIL.

Key to locations: t = top; c = centre; b = bottom; r = right; l = left; tr = top right; tl = top left; br = bottom right; bl = bottom left; cr = centre right; cl = centre left. (No abbreviation is given for pages with one image, or pages on which all images are by one photographer.

AB = Andy Belcher; CFPL = Chris Fairclough Picture Library; CC = Christel Clear; C-Map = C-Map South Africa; DPPI/HT = DPPI (Henri Thibault); GC = Gerald Cubitt; FN = Fotonatura; GI = Getty Images; IB = Image Bank (CC = Cosmo Condina; GC = Geoffrey Clifford; JK = John Kelly; PT = Paul Trummer); INPRA = INPRA; Kos = Kos (BG = Bob Grieser; CB = Carlo Borlenghi; GM = Gilles Martin-Raget); KS = K. Soehata; MF = Masterfile; NC = Neil Corder; NS = Neil Setchfield; NHIL = New Holland Image Library (NA = Nicholas Aldridge; PG = Peter Goldman); OI = Ocean Images; OW = Onne van der Wal; PG = Peter Goldman; PA = Photo Access (DWB = Dr Wagner/Bavaria; P = Pictor); PhotoB = Photo Bank (Peter Baker); PBPL = PictureBank Photo Library; PPL = PPL (AB = Alistair Black; AM = Adrian Morgan; BP = Barry Pickthall; DS = Dave Smyth; JLJ = Jamie Lawson-Johnston; JK = Jono Knight; RR = Roy Roberts); Ray = Raymarine; RHPL = Robert Harding Picture Library; RC = Richard Crocket; SA = Spade Anchor (Alain Poiraud); SIL = Struik Image Library (MC = Mike Carelse; RdlH = Roger de la Harpe); SL = Stefania Lamberti; TI = Travel Ink (AH = Angela Hampton); TM = courtesy of The Moorings.

Cover	main photo	Kos	52	l	NHIL/PG	110		CFPL
	tr	CC	53	tr	NC	111	l	PhotoB/PB
	2nd r	CC	54		PPL/AM	111	r	NS
	3rd r	NC	62		NC	112		RHPL
	br	PPL/DS	65		NC	113		TI/AH
	spine	FN	66	t	MF	114		PPL/DS
	back flap	RC	67	tr	SIL/MC	115		PPL/AB
	endpapers	NC	67	cr	NHIL/PG	116	l	NC
1		NC	67	br	CC	116	r	PBPL
4–5		NC	69	c	Ray	117		TM
6–7		TM	70	r	Ray	118		PPL/JK
8		TM	71	b	CC	119		PPL/JK
10	bl	PG	72		NC	120		PPL/AB
13	b	NC	74		NC	121		Kos/BG
14	bl	NC	75		GI	122	tr	Kos/CB
17		NC	81		NC	122	bl	IB/GC
22	bl	NC	86	tl	DPPI/HT	123		IB/CC
25		Kos/GM	88	l	AB	124		GC
31		NC	88	r	CC	125		SL
34		NC	89	l	OI	126		SIL/RdlH
37	2nd from top	NHIL/PG	90		INPRA	127		NC
37	b	SA/AP	94		PA/P	128		PPL
38		NC	96		PPL/BP	130		PPL/JLJ
40	tr	Ray	99		NC	131		NC
41	bl	CC	102		PhotoB/PB	132	br	NC
42		PPL	103		PA	133		NC
44		CC	104		NC	134		Kos/CB
45	b	Kos/GM	105		IB/JK	135		OW
47	br	NHIL/NA	106	tl	PhotoB/PB	136	l	PPL
50	tl	C-Map	106	br	PPL/AB	136	r	PPL/JK
50	bl	C-Map	107		NC	137		KS
50	tr	Ray	108	t	IB/PT	138		NC
50	br	Ray	108	bl	PPL/RR	139		NC
51	all	NHIL/NA	109		RHPL			

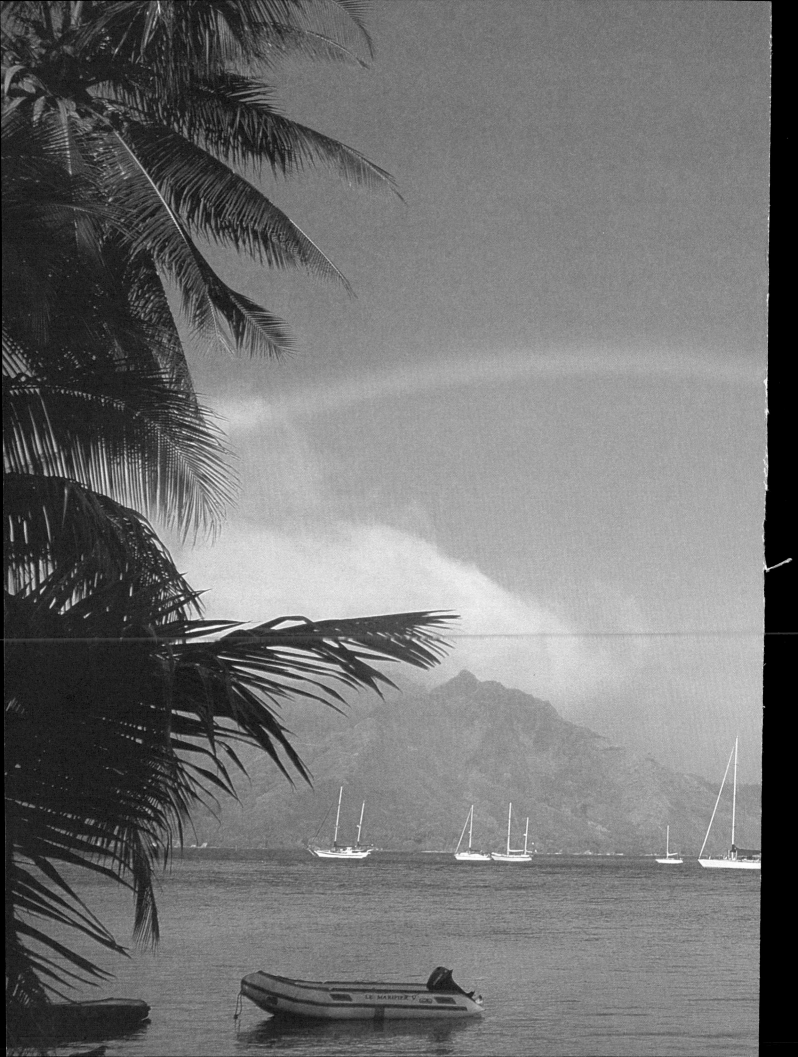